Quanbeck

To Dr. Lyle O. Johnston
and the Staff of the
Shriners Hospital in
Minneapolis, Mn.
    With best wishes,
            Ignacio V. Ponseti
        Sept. 98

Please return
to
Deb
Quanbeck

Congenital Clubfoot

Fundamentals of treatment

IGNACIO V. PONSETI

Professor Emeritus,
Department of Orthopaedic Surgery,
University of Iowa,
Iowa City, Iowa

Oxford   New York   Tokyo
OXFORD UNIVERSITY PRESS
1996

Oxford University Press, Walton Street, Oxford OX2 6DP

Oxford New York
Athens Auckland Bangkok Bombay
Calcutta Cape Town Dar es Salaám Delhi
Florence Hong Kong Istanbul Karachi
Kuala Lumpur Madras Madrid Melbourne
Mexico City Nairobi Paris Singapore
Taipei Tokyo Toronto
and associated companies in
Berlin Ibadan

Oxford is a trade mark of Oxford University Press

Published in the United States
by Oxford University Press Inc., New York

A catalogue record for this book is available from the British Library

Library of Congress Cataloging in Publication Data
Ponseti, I. V. (Ignacio V.), 1914–
Congenital clubfoot: fundamentals of treatment/Ignacio V. Ponseti.
Includes index.
1. Clubfoot.   I. Title. [DNLM: 1. Clubfoot–pathology.   2. Clubfoot–therapy. WE 883
P798c 1996]
RD783.P65 1996   617.5'85–dc20   96–13336

ISBN 0 19 262765 1 (h/b)

Typeset by EXPO Holdings, Malaysia

Printed in Great Britain by
Bookcraft (Bath) Ltd
Midsomer Norton, Avon

To my wife Helena Percas, Ph.D.
whose encouragement and generosity
has made this book possible

Preface

A new form of manipulative treatment of the congenital clubfoot was started in 1948 at the University of Iowa Hospitals. Our treatment, supported by limited operative interventions and based on a clear understanding of the functional anatomy of the foot, has yielded optimum results in a high percentage of patients, as attested by Drs Cooper and Dietz (1995) in a recent review of our patients treated 25 to 42 years ago. Although the treated clubfeet are less supple than normal feet, there are no significant differences in the functional performance of our patients compared to a population of similar age born with normal feet.

The purpose of this book is to explain why an orthopedic treatment—which takes advantage of the biological response of young connective tissue and bone to corrective position changes gradually obtained by manipulation and casting—is the sensible approach to the treatment of the congenital clubfoot. Joint releases and bone surgery should be used only in infrequent cases of very severe clubfeet with stiff tarsal ligaments unyielding to stretching.

In this book, therefore, I will present the gross and microscopic anatomy of the structures of the clubfoot in fetuses and stillborn babies to illustrate the basic anomalies of the deformity (Chapters 2 and 3). The functional anatomy of the normal foot, essential to the understanding of the treatment of the clubfoot deformity, is reviewed in Chapter 4. The pathogenesis of the clubfoot, based on recent biological research, is discussed in Chapter 5. Chapter 6 is devoted to the clinical history and examination of the patient. Chapter 7 is devoted to the manipulative treatment of the clubfoot followed by description of the few surgical interventions we perform. The results of our treatment in patients who were followed for many years and the radiographic study of the treated clubfeet are discussed in Chapters 9 and 10. Common errors and iatrogenic deformities and how to avoid them follows in Chapter 11.

It is my hope that orthopedists favoring radical early surgery, unaware that the bone, joint, and ligament deformities are largely reversible in the infant using the methods described in this book, will consider our approach to the treatment of clubfoot. This treatment is economical and easy on the baby and on the parents, and is in the best tradition of Orthopedia.

I am indebted to the many residents, fellows, and staff members who worked with me through the years on different aspects of clubfoot problems and the results of treatment; to Drs Eugene N. Smoley, Jerry. R. Becker, Jerónimo Campos, Sinesio Misol, Sterling J. Laaveg, Stuart L. Weinstein, Frederick R. Dietz, José M. Morcuende, and Douglas M. Cooper for their work in clinical research; to Dr Jerry Maynard for his studies of the leg muscles under the electron microscope; to Dr Victor Ionasescu for his studies of the protein synthesis in these muscles; to Dr Richard Brand for directing the work on foot kinematics; to Dr Georges Y. El-Khoury for his contribution in the roentgenological and computerized tomography studies; and to Dr Ernesto Ippolito, now professor at the University of Rome, for his important contribution to the pathology in clubfeet of fetuses. To all of them, I am profoundly grateful. Their close friendship engendered through collaborative work in our university setting has been one of the greatest rewards in my professional life.

Iowa City, US and Puerto Pollensa, Mallorca.　　　　　　　　　　I.V.P.
March 1996

References

Cooper, D.M. and Dietz, F.R. (1995). Treatment of idiopathic clubfoot. A thirty-year follow-up. *J. Bone Joint Surg. (Am.)*, **77A**, 1477.

Contents

1
Introduction

The clubfoot is one of the most common congenital deformities. Many cases are associated with neuromuscular diseases, chromosomal abnormalities, Mendelian and non-Mendelian syndromes, and in rare cases with extrinsic causes. In the present book, we are limiting ourselves to the study of the idiopathic congenital clubfoot deformity, occurring in otherwise normal infants. In Caucasians, the disorder occurs in about one per thousand; among the Japanese, it occurs half as frequently; in South African blacks it occurs three times as frequently; and in Polynesians it occurs six times as frequently. The ratio of male to female is 3 to 1, and 40 per cent of cases are bilateral (Chung *et al.* 1969; Yamamoto 1979; Cowell and Wein 1980; Cartlidge 1984; Yang *et al.* 1987).

The congenital clubfoot appears to be of genetic origin (Rebbeck *et al.* 1993). In a study based on 635 patients from Exeter, England, Ruth Wynne-Davies (1964*a,b*) calculated that if one child in a family has the deformity the chance of a second child having it is 1 in 35. Idelberger (1939) examined 174 pairs of twins with clubfoot. In 32.5 per cent (1 in 3) of identical (monozygotic) twins, both had clubfeet, whereas in only 2.9 per cent of fraternal twins (dizygotic), both had clubfeet. This latter figure of 2.9 per cent is the same as that found by Ruth Wynne-Davies for the incidence of non-twin siblings in Exeter.

Idiopathic congenital clubfoot may be associated with other congenital abnormalities. Metatarsus varus (adductus) was observed by Kite in 8 per cent of 764 patients with unilateral clubfoot (Kite 1930). In the 70 clubfoot patients studied by Laaveg and myself, 36 had unilateral clubfoot (Laaveg and Ponseti 1980). Eight of these (22.2 per cent) had metatarsus adductus, a higher incidence than reported by Kite. Among the 1200 clubfoot patients initially treated by me, I have estimated but not reported an incidence of metatarsus adductus in 18 per cent of the cases. Ruth Wynne-Davies (1964*a*) found joint laxity in 17 to 18 per cent of her patients, an incidence of hernia not higher than in the normal population, one child with congenital dislocation of the hip, and 4 to 5 per cent with other deformities in the limbs such as ring constrictions, syndactyly, and missing or extra fingers.

The pathology, the functional anatomy of clubfoot, and the structural changes in its ligaments, tendons, and muscles, must be well understood to arrive at a sound approach to early non-surgical treatment of this deformity. The congenital clubfoot is a complex three-dimensional deformity having four components: equinus, varus, adductus, and cavus. Since the definitions of foot movements and of movements of tarsal bones are confusing in the orthopedic literature, yet basic to the understanding of the deformity and its treatment, we shall describe the direction of rotation of a tarsal bone by the appropriately used terms of abduction/adduction, flexion/extension, and inversion/eversion. In agreement with the international SFTR method, we define these terms according to Russe and Gerhard (1975), as reported by Van Langelaan (1983; Fig. 1).

- adduction is that movement of a tarsal bone in which the distal part of this bone moves towards the median body plane;
- abduction is this movement in the opposite direction;
- flexion is that movement of a tarsal bone in which the distal part of that bone moves in the plantar direction;

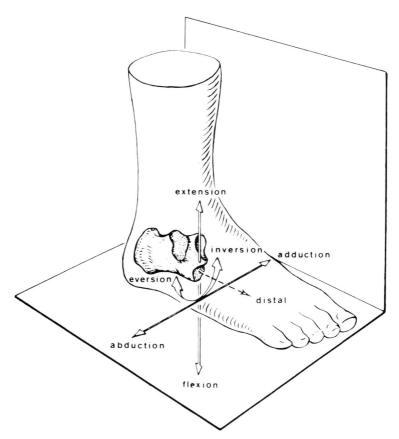

Fig. 1 Definitions of movements for a tarsal (calcaneal) bone with respect to the body planes. (From Van Langelaan 1983.)

- extension is the movement in the opposite direction;
- inversion is the movement of a tarsal bone in which the undersurface of the bone moves towards the median body plane;
- eversion is the movement in the opposite direction.

We reserve the term supination for combined movements of adduction, flexion, and inversion, and the term pronation for combined movements of abduction, extension, and eversion.

The term heel varus is used for movements of inversion and adduction of the calcaneus, and the term heel valgus is used for eversion and abduction of the calcaneus.

The term forefoot supination is used for movements of inversion and adduction of the forepart of the foot and the term forefoot pronation is used for eversion and abduction of the forepart of the foot.

Equinus refers to an increased degree of plantar flexion of the foot.

Cavus refers to the increased height of the vault of the foot.

The treatment of clubfoot has been controversial throughout the last 150 years. When I arrived in the University of Iowa Medical School to complete my training in orthopedic surgery in 1941, the clubfoot was treated by different members of the staff, some with manipulations and plaster casts, others by taping the feet in Denis Browne splints, and still others by using the Kite's (1930) method: removing some wedges from a plaster shoe to correct the components of the deformity. The Thomas wrench was occasionally used to correct residual deformities but finally most feet ended up in surgery. The Brockman technique for the medial release of the subtalar and midtarsal joints was one of the most common operations performed in the department (Brockman 1930). My colleagues and I expanded the medial release operation to include a posterior release and often we made a lateral incision to free the tarsal joints so as to align the tarsal bones with the cuneiforms and metatarsals (Le Noir 1966). Most often this surgery left deep scarring, joint stiffness and weakness. The techniques of treatment and results in our department before 1948 were reported by Steindler, Le Noir, and others (Blumenfeld *et al.* 1946; Steindler 1950, 1955; Le Noir 1966).

Robert Jones from Liverpool and London wrote in 1923 that he had 'never met with a case where treatment has been started in the first week where the deformity could not be completely rectified by manipulation and retention in two months' (Jones 1923). His experience could not be duplicated in our department nor in other clinics I visited, and the results were far from perfect after a very prolonged treatment. Faced with these disappointing results, I set out to discover how a clubfoot could be corrected through manipulation and retention casts in a two-month period after birth, as Robert Jones had claimed.

Although Kite was the leading advocate of the conservative treatment of clubfoot for many years and should be commended for his lifetime efforts to try to resolve the clubfoot problem without surgery, his treatment was lengthy and short of satisfactory. I was determined to discover the flaws that prevented him from reaching Robert Jones's claimed results. In 1960, I visited Kite in Atlanta for a few days to observe his method of treatment. In 1965, we gave a course together in Caracas, Venezuela, during which each of us applied plaster casts. Our methods differed greatly.

Kite corrected each component of the deformity separately instead of simultaneously, and although he managed to correct the cavus and to avoid foot pronation and its harmful consequences, the correction of the heel varus took him an inordinate amount of time since he did not realize that the calcaneus must abduct before it can be everted. However, he managed to obtain plantigrade feet. I shall go into further detail in Chapter 7 where I discuss the manipulative treatment.

From my observations in the clinic and in the operating room, I realized that the orthopedists' failures in the treatment of clubfoot were related, in part, to a poor understanding of the functional anatomy of the normal foot as well as of the clubfoot. Without this understanding, it is impossible to alter the forces that caused the deformity and apply the proper corrective manipulations and retaining casts. I then studied the pathological anatomy of the clubfoot. I dissected several normal feet and three clubfeet of stillborn babies, and obtained serial sections of the two clubfeet of a 17-week aborted fetus. Under cineradiography, I studied the range of motions of the tarsal joints of normal feet and of clubfeet. I trained my fingers to palpate the joints and bones and feel their motions both in normal feet and in clubfeet.

Based on these studies, I developed and refined a uniform type of treatment in the late forties. By the late fifties, when reviewing our patients for a short-term follow-up article (Ponseti and Smoley 1963), I knew that I had found the proper approach to the treatment of clubfoot, a treatment that has been followed to the present day in our department with optimum results. Fellows joining our pediatric orthopedic program were impressed to discover the ease with which most clubfeet can be well corrected without surgery in a relatively short time in contrast to the poorer results experienced in other hospitals after extensive manipulations and surgeries. Although relapses were frequent, usually two years after treatment, most could be successfully treated with further manipulations and castings for four to six weeks or with a transfer of the tibialis anterior tendon in severe cases.

Many orthopedic specialists, however, choose surgery over manipulation as the best treatment for clubfeet. This view explains the disappointing results obtained after prolonged faulty manipulations and casting, usually carried out by assistants not thoroughly acquainted with the complexities of the deformity. To correct the severe supination the clubfoot is forcefully pronated instead of abducted. These manipulations cause an increase of the cavus and severe distortions in the tarsal joints and midfoot, making further treatment, whether manipulative or surgical, very difficult or impossible.

The biological anomalies in congenital clubfoot have not been studied in great depth. Many orthopedists dealing with clubfoot lack an understanding of the nature of its anatomy and kinematics and of the pathology of the clubfoot's ligaments, tendons and muscles, although such an understanding is crucial for the treatment of this deformity. This lack of understanding has led to major errors in treatment. Most publications on the subject deal with a large variety of surgical interventions under the mistaken assumption that early alignment of the displaced skeletal elements results in a normal anatomy of bones, joints, ligaments, capsules, and muscles, as well as the mistaken assumptions that roentgenographic appearance in early ages relates to long-term function, and that joint capsules and ligaments can be stripped away and tendons can be lengthened with impunity. These misconceptions have resulted in poor corrections, much suffering, and a number of iatrogenic deformities. In a recent publication (Simons 1994) of the papers presented at a congress on clubfeet, there are scores of reports on surgical procedures, many of them untested, and some exclusively designed for telcome datacomphe treatment of iatrogenic deformities. The chapters in that publication on complications of clubfoot surgery attest to the tragic failures of early surgery.

An immediate surgical correction of the clubfoot components is anatomically impossible. After extensive dissections to release joint capsules and ligaments and to lengthen tendons, the tarsal joints do not match. In order to hold the bones roughly in proper alignment, the surgeon is forced to transfix them with wires. Stripping the joint capsules and ligaments, and lengthening tendons cause joint damage, stiffness, overcorrections or undercorrections, and muscle weakness. Long-term functional results of these operations have not been published. In my experience many clubfeet treated surgically become stiff and painful after the second decade of life. The numerous clinical and roentgenographic measurements used to evaluate treatment are subjective in nature and are not always reproducible. In addition, results before completion of skeletal maturity do not foretell long-term functional outcomes (Laaveg and Ponseti 1980; Cummings *et al*. 1994).

A well-conducted orthopedic treatment, based on a sound understanding of the functional anatomy of the foot and on the biological response of young connective tissue and bone to changes in direction of mechanical stimuli, can gradually reduce or almost eliminate these deformities in most clubfeet. Less than 5 per cent of infants with very severe, short, fat feet with stiff ligaments unyielding to stretching will need surgical correction. The parents of all the other infants may be reassured that their baby, when treated by expert hands, will have a functional, plantigrade foot which is normal in appearance, requires no special shoes, and allows fairly good mobility.

The guidelines for the clubfoot method of treatment which I developed in 1948, described in full detail in Chapter 7, are as follows:

1. All the components of the clubfoot deformity have to be corrected simultaneously with the exception of the equinus which should be corrected last.
2. The cavus, which results from a pronation of the forefoot in relation to the hindfoot, is corrected as the foot is abducted by supinating the forefoot and thereby placing it in proper alignment with the hindfoot.

3. While the whole foot is held in supination and in flexion, it can be gently and gradually abducted under the talus secured against rotation in the ankle mortice by applying counter-pressure with the thumb against the lateral aspect of the head of the talus.

4. The heel varus and foot supination will correct when the entire foot is fully abducted in maximum external rotation under the talus. The foot should never be everted.

5. Now the equinus can be corrected by dorsiflexing the foot. The tendo Achilles may need to be subcutaneously sectioned to facilitate this correction.

The same guidelines are applied in the initial treatment of the severe, rigid clubfeet in patients with arthrogryposis and myelomeningoceles. In these infants, however, the deformity may be more difficult or even impossible to correct satisfactorily. Any improvement in the alignment obtained is usually lost shortly after the plaster cast is removed. Relapses occur even after extensive tarsal joint releases. In these severe deformities talectomy after one year of age is the best operation to obtain plantigrade feet, albeit with defficient function.

References

Blumenfeld, I., Kaplan, M., and Hicks, E.O. (1946). The conservative treatment for congenital talipes equinovarus. *J. Bone Joint Surg.*, **28**, 765.

Brockman, F.P. (1930). *Congenital club foot.* John Wright, Bristol, and Simpkin Marshall, London.

Cartlidge, I. (1984). Observations on the epidemiology of club foot in Polynesian and Caucasian populations. *J. Med. Genet.*, **21**, 290.

Chung, C.S., Nemechek, R.W., Larsen, I.J., and Ching, G.H.S. (1969). Genetic and epideminological study of clubfoot in Hawaii. *Hum. Hered.*, **19**, 321.

Cowell, H.R. and Wein, B.K. (1980). Genetic aspects of clubfoot. *J. Bone Joint Surg.*, **62A**, 1381.

Cummings, R.J., Hay, R.M., McCluskey, W.P., Mazur, J.M., and Lovell, W.W. (1994). Can clubfeet be evaluated accurately and reproducibly? In *The clubfoot* (ed. G.W. Simons). Springer-Verlag, New York.

Idelberger, K. (1939). Die Ergebnisse der Zwillingsforschung beim angeborenen Klumpfuss. *Verhandlungen der Deutschen Orthopaedischen Gesellschaft*, **33**, 272.

Jones, R. (1923). The treatment of clubfoot in the newly born. *Lancet*, **1**, 713.

Kite, J.H. (1930). Non-operative treatment of congenital clubfeet. *Southern Med. J.*, **23**, 337.

Laaveg, S.J. and Ponseti, I.V. (1980). Long term results of treatment of congenital club foot. *J. Bone Joint Surg.*, **62A**, 23.

LeNoir, J. (1966). *Congenital idiopathic talipes.* Charles C. Thomas, Springfield, IL.

Ponseti, I.V. and Smoley, E.N. (1963). Congenital club foot: The results of treatment. *J. Bone Joint Surg.*, **45A**, 261.

Rebbeck, T.R., Dietz, F.R., Murray, J.C., and Buetow, K.H. (1993). A single gene explanation for the probability of having Idiopathic Talipes equinovarus. *Am. J. Hum. Genet.*, **53**, 1051.

Simons, G.W. (ed.) (1994). *The clubfoot.* Springer–Verlag, New York.

Steindler, A (1950). *Post-graduate lectures on orthopaedic diagnosis and indications.* Charles C. Thomas, Springfield, IL.

Steindler, A (1955). *Kinesiology of the human body.* Charles C. Thomas, Springfield, IL.

Van Langelaan, E.J. (1983). A kinematical analysis of the tarsal joints. *Acta Orthop. Scand.*, **54** (Suppl. 204), 135.

Wynne-Davies, R. (1964*a*). Family studies and cause of congenital clubfoot. *J. Bone Joint Surg.*, **46B**, 445.

Wynne-Davies, R. (1964*b*). Talipes equinovarus. A review of eighty-four cases after completion of treatment. *J. Bone Joint Surg.*, **46B**, 464.

Yamamoto, H. (1979). A clinical, genetic and epidemiological study of congenital clubfoot. *Jpn J. Hum. Genet.*, **24**, 37.

Yang, H., Chung, C.S., and Nemechek, R.W. (1987). A genetic analysis of clubfoot in Hawaii. *Genet. Epidemiol.*, **4**, 299.

2
Pathological anatomy

The abnormal anatomy of the congenital clubfoot was well described by Antonio Scarpa (1803) in his *Memoria chirurgica sui piedi torti congeniti*. He noted the medial displacement and inversion (turned around their shorter axes) of the navicular, of the cuboid, and of the calcaneus in relation to the talus. He believed that the anomalies of the muscles, tendons, and ligaments of the foot and leg were secondary to the skeletal deformity.

In his book, *Club-foot, its causes, pathology and treatment*, first published in 1866, William Adams (1973) described his findings on thirty clubfeet and concluded that the main anomaly resides in the medial and plantar deflection of the neck and head of the talus and that this anomaly was 'an adaptation to the altered position of the os calcis and scafoid, being the result rather than the cause of the deformity'.

Following these classical works there appeared a large number of publications on the abnormal anatomy of the clubfoot. Some forty scientifically reliable studies were based on anatomical studies of clubfeet in fetuses, and in untreated stillborn or deceased infants (Bissell 1888; Virchow 1933; Bechtol and Mossman 1950; Irani and Sherman 1963; Schlicht 1963; Settle 1963; Hjelmstedt and Sahlstedt 1974; Howard and Benson 1993). The numerous publications based upon casual anatomical observations made in the operating room in the course of clubfoot surgery are often unreliable and even misleading.

The anatomy of the clubfoot is best understood by studying fetuses of different ages and babies after birth. Since 1947, we have studied serial histological sections of twelve clubfeet and four normal feet of four fetuses with bilateral deformities and four fetuses with unilateral deformities; all the fetuses were aborted at 16 to 24 weeks of gestation. These studies were complemented with anatomical dissections of three clubfeet of stillborn babies and three clubfeet recovered from two full-term babies dead shortly after birth; one of the latter had bilateral deformity and the other had unilateral.

A complete postmortem examination of the fetuses, including the central nervous system in three, revealed no abnormalities other than the clubfoot. Oligohydramnios was not observed in any of the cases. The spinal cord of one fetus was sectioned serially for histological examination and was found to be normal. The legs of four fetuses with bilateral clubfeet were disarticulated at the knee while the legs of the other fetuses were severed at the mid-point between the knee and the ankle. The histological sections in the normal feet and clubfeet of the fetuses were cut approximately in the sagittal, frontal, and transverse planes. Since a clubfoot is deformed in three dimensions, often it is impossible to obtain exactly similar cuts from normal and clubfeet for comparison. Three clubfeet of fetuses 17 to 20 weeks of age were sectioned in the frontal plane of the leg and ankle mortice.

The specimens were fixed, decalcified, and embedded in paraffin. Serial sections were stained, some with hematoxylin and eosin; some with alcian blue, periodic acid–Schiff, and Weigert hematoxylin; and others with Masson trichrome. The morphological features of the clubfeet and of the normal feet as observed in each plane were described only after a complete study of all the serial sections was done to obtain a clear understanding of the spatial arrangements of the structures of the foot. The sizes of the muscles and of the muscle fibers and the amount of connective tissue in the muscles, fasciae, and tendons in the sections of the middle and lower thirds of the leg were compared in trichrome-stained sections of the normal limbs and of the limbs with clubfeet, and any differences were estimated.

An autopsy was performed in the two full-term infants, one dead at birth from asphyxia, with unilateral clubfoot, and the other with bilateral clubfeet dead from a congenital heart defect at three days of age. No other defects were observed in the musculoskeletal or central nervous systems. The clubfeet and the normal foot were dissected. The bones, joints, muscles, tendons, and igaments were carefully studied.

A seventeen-week-old fetus obtained when the mother died in a car accident had bilateral clubfoot, mild on the right and severe on the left (Fig. 2). Serial sec-

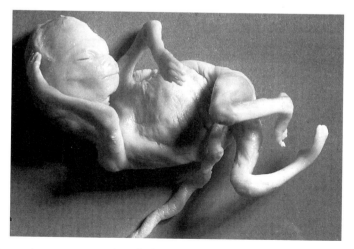

Fig. 2 90-mm (crown to rump) male (17-week-old fetus) with bilateral clubfoot, mild on the right, severe on the left.

tions were made of both feet and both legs in the frontal plane of the ankle. Owing to the supination and adduction deformity of both feet, the sections of the middle and anterior aspects of the two feet were in a very oblique plane.

In the left foot the navicular was medially displaced and its tuberosity was very close to the medial malleolus (Fig. 3B). The navicular was wedge-shaped so that its lateral and plantar surfaces were narrow. There were three fairly well developed articulations between the talus and the calcaneus. The tendon of the tibialis posterior was very large and its sheath was very thick (Fig. 3F). The tibionavicular and calcanonavicular ligaments were very thick and short and very cellular (Fig. 3D). The deep layer of the deltoid ligament was thick and appeared to have been pulled into the joint between the medial malleolus and the talus (Fig. 3D). The talocalcaneal interosseus ligament in the sinus tarsi was formed by thin strands of collagen fibers that were nearly devoid of cells.

In the right foot the navicular was of nearly normal shape and was less medially displaced than the navicular in the left foot (Fig. 3A). The heel was displaced into a varus position and the foot was supinated (Figs 3A, 3C, and 3E). All tendons and tendon sheaths were of nearly normal size except that the tendon of the tibialis posterior was very thick at its insertion (Fig. 3E). The tibionavicular and calcaneonavicular ligaments were thick but the other ligaments were of nearly normal thickness and length (Fig. 3C). The deep layer of the deltoid ligament was interposed between the medial malleolus and the talus (Figs 3C and 3E).

In both feet there was dense fibrous tissue located between the calcaneus and the navicular which resembled a fibrous calcaneonavicular bar (Fig. 3A and 3B).

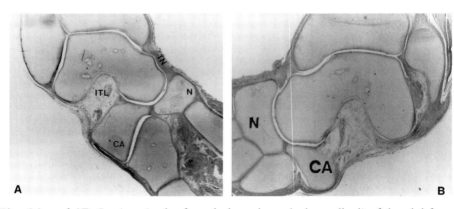

Figs 3A and 3B Sections in the frontal plane through the malleoli of the clubfeet of the fetus in Fig. 2. The right foot (A) is slightly supinated and adducted. At this level the tibionavicular ligament (TN) is slightly thickened (hematoxylin and eosin, × 9). The left foot (B) is in severe supination and adduction. The tibionavicular ligament (TN) is short and thick. The navicular (N) is slightly wedge-shaped laterally (hematoxylin and erosin, × 10). There is dense fibrous tissue, between the navicular and the anterior process of the calcaneus in both feet, possibly the fetal stage of a calcaneonavicular bar.

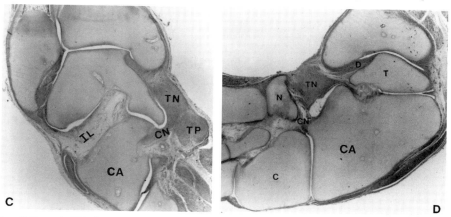

Fig. 3C and 3D In sections posterior to those shown in Fig. 3A and B, the deep layer of the deltoid ligament in both feet seems to have been pulled in between the talus and the medial malleolus. The tibionavicular ligament (TN) is very thick and shorter on the left (D) than on the right (C) and merges with the short plantar calcaneonavicular ligament (CN). In the right foot (C) the tibialis posterior tendon (TP) is very thick. The interosseous talocalcaneal ligament (IL) is thin and loose (hematoxylin and eosin, × 10). CA = calcaneus, C = cuboid.

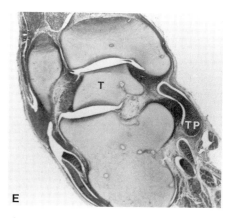

Fig. 3E In a section of the right foot posterior to that shown in Fig. 3C, the talo-alcaneal joint is seen to be well developed. The deep layer of the deltoid ligament is very thick and appears to have been pulled in between the medial malleolus and the talus (T). The tibialis posterior tendon (TP) is large. (Masson trichrome, × 10).

In all clubfeet, the talus was in severe flexion. The body of the talus was small and altered in shape. Usually the trochlea height was decreased. The anterior part of the trochlea was in some cases broader and in other cases of the same width as the posterior part. Only the posterior part of the trochlea articulated with the ankle mortice. The anterior part was covered by the

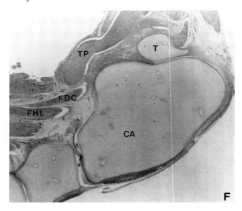

Fig. 3F In a section posterior to that shown in Fig. 3D, the foot appears to be in severe varus position and only the posterior tubercle of the talus (T) is seen, whereas the calcaneus (CA) is cut in a plane that extends its full length. The tibialis posterior tendon (TP) is much thicker than the tendons of the flexor digitorum communis (FDC) and the flexor hallucis longus (FHL), nearly of normal size (hematoxylin and eosin, × 10).

stretched and thin anterior capsule of the ankle joint. In severe cases, the posterior surfaces of the lower end of both the tibia and the fibula were in contact with the superior aspect of the posterior tuberosity of the calcaneus. (Figs 4A and 4B) Therefore, the posterior part of the body of the talus, which was not covered by joint cartilage, was intra-articular. In one severe case, the talus was slightly inverted in the ankle mortice. The neck of the talus was medially and plantarly deflected. The head was wedge-shaped. There were two surfaces on the talar head: the anterolateral surface, left uncovered by the displaced navicular, was covered only by the stretched joint capsule and the skin; the anteromedial surface extended over the inner surface of the neck and articulated with the navicular (Fig. 7B).

The navicular was uniformly flattened or laterally wedge-shaped and severely medially displaced, adducted, and inverted. The medial tuberosity was large and very close to the medial malleolus; it presented a wide area for the insertion of the enlarged tibialis posterior tendon. This tendon also had a wide insertion in the plantar surface of the first cuneiform (Figs 7A, 7B, and 7C).

The body of the calcaneus was consistently in severe flexion and slightly medially bowed. In some cases it was of the same length and in others it was longer than the calcaneus of the normal controls. The calcaneus was adducted and inverted underneath the talus, and most of the anterior tuberosity of the calcaneus was under the head of the talus and not lateral to it as it is in normal feet. The longitudinal axes of the talus and the calcaneus were parallel. The cuboid was medially displaced and inverted in front of the calcaneus. Only the medial part of the anterior tuberosity of the calcaneus articulated with the cuboid (Fig. 8).

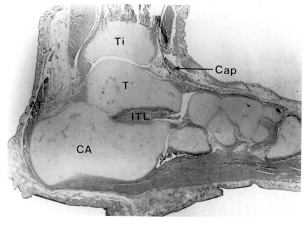

A

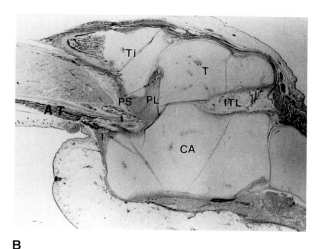

B

Fig. 4A and 4B Normal right foot of a 20-week-old fetus (Fig. 4A) and right club-foot of a 19-week-old fetus (Fig. 4B), sectioned in the sagittal plane through the middle of the ankle joint.

In (Fig. 4B) the tibia (Ti) articulates only with the most posterior part of the trochlea of the talus (T). The posterior fibulotalar and posterior talocalcaneal ligaments (PL) are pulled forward between the non-articular posterior surface of the talus and the inferior articular surface of the tibia and are matted together with the posterior ligament (PS) of the inferior tibiofibular syndesmosis. The tendo Achilles (AT) is tight and has a tri-angular-shaped insertion (I) into the posterior tuberosity of the calcaneus. The interosseous talocalcaneal ligament (ITL) in the sinus tarsi is thin and loose-textured. The number and distribution of the vascular channels in the talus is similar in both feet (hematoxylin and eosin, × 7).

The cuneiforms and metatarsals were always adducted but were normal in shape. The extent to which the relationships of the skeletal components were altered ranged from mild to severe and was better seen in some planes of section than in others.

The talocalcaneal articulations were very abnormal. The anterior joint was very narrow or absent, whereas the middle varied in size. In some feet the middle joint covered only a very small area of the sustentaculum tali (Fig. 5). In other feet the middle joint was large and in one foot it joined the posterior joint. The posterior joint in the sagittal plane was short and in the frontal plane it was horizontal in some cases and laterally inclined in other cases. In the most severe cases, the posterior joint extended only to the middle of the inferior surface of the talus, and to the corresponding middle part of the superior surface of the calcaneus. The lateral parts of these surfaces were not articulated and were not covered by articular cartilage even in the early stages of fetal life. Similarly, in one case the trochlea of the talus had articular cartilage only in its medial and posterior parts. Otherwise, in most subluxated joints, the articular cartilage of the non-articulating areas was morphologically and histochemically normal.

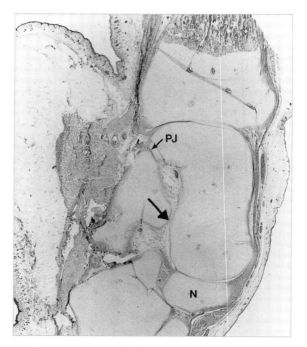

Fig. 5 Right clubfoot of a 19-week-old fetus sectioned in the sagittal plane through the ankle and the posterior and middle subtalar joints. The posterior subtalar joint (PJ) is very small and at the site of the middle subtalar joint (*arrow*) there is loose connective tissue and no joint capsule. The most lateral part of the navicular (N) is included in the section (hematoxylin and eosin, × 7).

Areolar tissue with many blood vessels filled the gap between the non-articulating surfaces. We observed no adhesions between the capsules and the joint surfaces. Fibrosis and adhesions of the joint capsules and ossification in non-articular cartilage, however, have been described in clubfeet dissected in late fetal life and after birth as well (Hjelmstedt and Sahlstedt 1974).

In the ankle, the tendons of the tibialis anterior, extensor digitorum longus, and extensor hallucis longus were severely displaced medially (Figs 6A and 6B). The tendon of the tibialis posterior was very large and further enlarged down to its insertion. All the ligaments of the inferior tibiofibular syndesmosis were very thick. The posterior ligament often formed a fibrotic mass matted together with the posterior fibulotalar and the posterior talocalcaneal ligaments. (Figs 6A and 6B) Fibrous tissue from the deep layer of the deltoid ligament was located between the contiguous surfaces of the medial malleolus and the medial articular facet of the talus (Hjelmstedt and Sahlstedt 1974).

In our specimens, some of the ligaments and capsules of the affected joints appeared to have become adapted to the altered joint positions because they were folded or stretched, whereas other ligaments were greatly shortened and thickened. The medial talocalcaneal ligament was markedly thickened. The anterior part of the deltoid ligament and the plantar calcaneonavicular ligament were short and thick in all the clubfeet we examined. In many cases they were

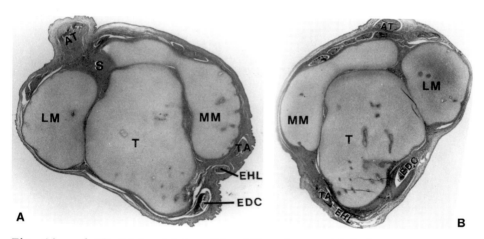

Fig. 6A and 6B Right clubfoot (Fig. 6A) and normal left foot (Fig. 6B) of a 16-week-old fetus: comparable sections in the transverse plane through the body and neck of the talus (T). Comparing the two feet, the following changes are seen in the club foot. The body of the talus is small and misshapen and the neck is medially angulated; the tibialis anterior (TA), extensor hallucis longus (EHL), and extensor digitorum communis (EDC) tendons are severely medially displaced; the deep layer of the deltoid ligament is interposed between the medial facet of the talus and the medial malleolus (MM); the ligaments of the inferior tibiofibular syndesmosis (S) are very thick; and the tendo achillis (AT) is large and hypertrophic at this level (hematoxylin and eosin, × 4.25).

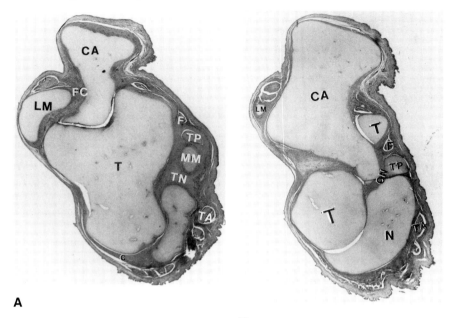

A

B

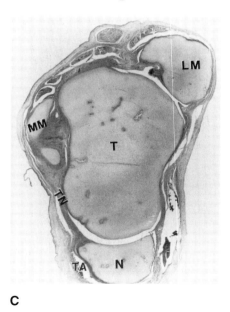

C

Fig. 7A, 7B, and 7C Right clubfoot (Figs 7A and 7B) and normal left foot (Fig. 7C) of a 16-week-old fetus, sectioned in the transverse plane through the talonavicular joint. Figures 7A and 7C are sections through the tip of the medial malleolus (MM) of both limbs. In the clubfoot (Fig. 7A), the section passes through both the talus (T) and the calcaneus (CA), but in the normal foot (Fig. 7C) the cut passes through the talus and above the calcaneus. Figure 7B is a more distal section through the tip of the lateral malleolus (LM) of the limb with the clubfoot.

In the clubfoot (Fig. 7A) the navicular (N) is medially subluxated and its tuberosity is close to the medial malleolus. The lateral part of the capsule (C) of the talonavicular joint is stretched, whereas the tibionavicular ligament (TN) is very thick and short The tibialis posterior tendon (TP) is thick and has a wide insertion on the tuberosity of the navicular, where it contains an area of hyaline cartilage (Fig. 7B). The sheath of the tibialis posterior tendon is thick and the plantar calcaneonavicular ligament (CN), is short. The fibulocalcaneal ligament (FC) is also thick and short. The number and distribution of the vascular channels in the body and head of the talus are similar in both feet. The navicular is elongated and its lateral part is flat. The tibialis anterior tendon (TA) is displaced medially (hematoxylin and eosin, × 10).

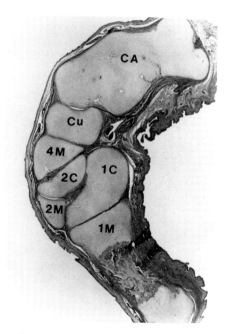

Fig. 8 Right clubfoot of 16-week-old fetus sectioned in the transverse plane through the calcaneocuboid joint. The cuboid (Cu) is medially subluxated on the calcaneus (CA), which appears bowed so that it is concave medially. In front of the cuboid is the base of the fourth metatarsal (4M) and medial to this are the second (2C) and first (1C) cuneiforms. The first metatarsal (1M) and the base of the second metatarsal (2M) are in front of the first and second cuneiforms, respectively. The first metatarsal articulates with the first cuneiform. The tendons of the flexor digitorum longus and flexor hallucis longus are medial to the cuboid (hematoxylin and eosin, × 6).

distorted and matted together with the adjoining tendon sheaths. The posterior tibiotalar, the fibulotalar, and the fibulocalcaneal ligaments were also thick and short and often matted together with abundant fibrous tissue. In the very severe cases, the ligaments of the posterior aspect of the ankle joint were pulled into the joint and their insertions on the talus were covered by the articular surface of the tibia (Fig. 4B).

The interosseous talocalcaneal ligaments in the sinus tarsi were under-developed and often consisted of a few connective tissue strands. This was observed even in the older specimens. The bifurcate ligament was stretched and thin. The calcaneocuboid ligaments and the navicular cuneiform ligaments were normal or only slightly enlarged, and the ligaments in the forefoot and toes were of normal thickness. The plantar fascia was thick in only three fetuses.

The morphological changes observed in the six clubfeet studied at birth were similar to the changes observed in the fetuses. The talus, although in severe equinus, was firmly fitted in the ankle mortise. The greatest distortion was seen in the navicular, which was severely medially displaced, inverted, and articulated with the medial aspect of the head of the talus which was wedge-shaped. The navicular tuberosity was nearly in contact with the tip of the medial malleolus. The inversion of the navicular appeared to be caused by the

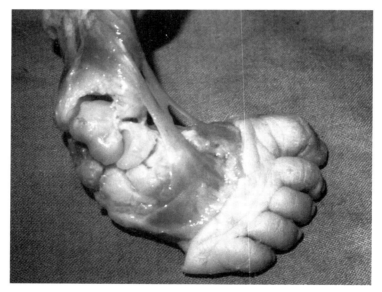

Fig. 9A Clubfoot of a 3-day-old infant. The navicular is medially displaced and articulates only with the medial aspect of the head of the talus. The cuneiforms are seen to the right of the navicular and the cuboid is underneath it. The calcaneocuboid joint is directed posteromedially. The anterior two-thirds of the os calcis is seen underneath the talus. The tendons of the tibialis anterior, extensor hallucis longus, and extensor digitorum longus are medially displaced.

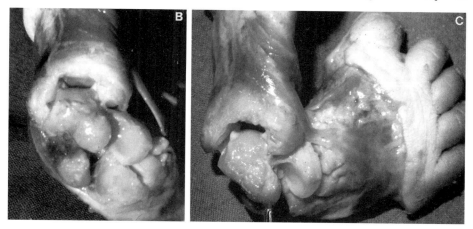

Figs 9B and 9C (9B) The anterior tuberosity of the calcaneous and (9C) the head of the talus are wedge-shaped and would not match with the joint surfaces of the cuboid and the navicular if a surgical reduction were attempted.

retraction of the deltoid and spring ligaments and by the traction of the short-ened tibialis posterior tendon which inserts in the lower part of the navicular tuberosity and first cuneiform and gives off fibrous expansion to the other cuneiforms and to the cuboid. The inversion varied from 40 degrees in the milder cases to 80 degrees in severe ones. Thus, the position of the navicular changes from horizontal in the normal foot to nearly vertical in the severe clubfoot. All the medial tarsal ligaments and the posterior tibial tendon and tendon sheath were greatly thickened and enlarged (Figs 9A, 9B, and 9C).

The calcaneus was adducted underneath the talus. There was a gap filled with fibrous tissue in the lateral aspect of the subtalar joint with a large opening of the sinus tarsi. Just as is found in fetuses, the posterior talocalcaneal joint was small in size and, although nearly horizontal in the back it was inclined laterally in front. The medial talocalcaneal joint was small and the anterior joint was absent. In clubfeet of neonates, Howard and Benson (1993) have observed the medial facet of the calcaneus to lie vertically, so that with the inverted cal-caneus, the subtalar joint is sagittally rather than coronally oriented. In the infants we studied the cuboid (Fig. 9B) was adducted and inverted in front of the wedge-shaped anterior joint surface of the calcaneus. The cuneiforms and the metatarsals were adducted but of normal shape. In some cases, however, the anterior joint surface of the first cuneiform was slanted medially. As in the fetuses, the tendons of the anterior tibial, extensor hallucis longus, and extensor digitorum longus were medially displaced over and just in front of the medial malleolus.

The inversion and adduction of the calcaneus accounted for the varus deformity of the heel. The heel varus, and the adduction and inversion of the navicular and cuboid, accounted for the supination of the clubfoot. The skeletal components of the anterior part of the foot were adducted in front of the severely medially displaced navicular and cuboid. The first metatarsal was in more flexion than the lateral metatarsals, and this accounted for the cavus. The long plantar ligaments were not or were only slightly hypertrophic.

References

Adams, W. (1973). *Club-foot. Its causes pathology and treatment*, (2nd edn), Lindsay & Blakiston, Philadelphia.

Bechtol, C.O. and Mossman, H.W. (1950). Club-foot. An embryological study of associated muscle abnormalities. *J. Bone Joint Surg.*, **32A**, 827.

Bissell, J.B. (1888). The morbid anatomy of congenital talipes equinovarus. *Arch. Pediatr.*, **5**, 406.

Hjelmstedt, A. and Sahlstedt, B. (1974). Talar deformity in congenital clubfeet. An anatomical and functional study with special reference to the ankle joint mobility. *Acta Orthop. Scand.*, **45**, 628.

Howard, C.B. and Benson, M.K.D. (1933). Clubfoot: Its pathological anatomy. *J. Pediat. Orthop.*, **13**, 654.

Irani, R.N. and Sherman, M.S. (1963). The pathological anatomy of clubfoot. *J. Bone Joint Surg.*, **45A**, 45.

Scarpa, A. (1803). *Memoria chirurgica sui piedi torti congeniti dei fanciu e sulla maniera di correggere questa deformita*. Pavia.

Schlicht, D. (1963). The pathological anatomy of talipes equinovarus. *Aust. N.Z. J. Surg.*, **33**, 1.

Settle, G.W. (1963). The anatomy of congenital talipes equinovarus: Sixteen dissected specimens. *J. Bone Joint Surg.*, **45A**, 1341.

Virchow, H. (1933). Klumpfusse nach Form zusammengesetzt. *Arch. Orthop. Unfallchir.*, **33**, 324.

3
Structural changes of muscles, tendons, and ligaments of the leg and foot

Muscles

The muscle-tendon unit of the triceps surae and of the tibialis posterior is smaller and shorter in the clubfoot than in the normal foot (Fig. 10). In the

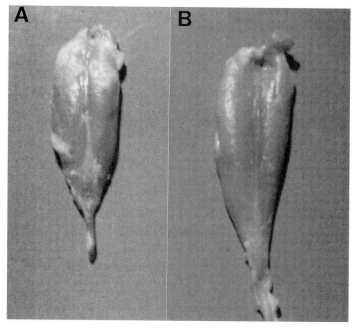

Fig. 10 Gastrocnemius muscles from a 6-month-old premature baby with unilateral clubfoot. The muscle of the leg with the clubfoot (A) is smaller than the muscle in the normal side (B).

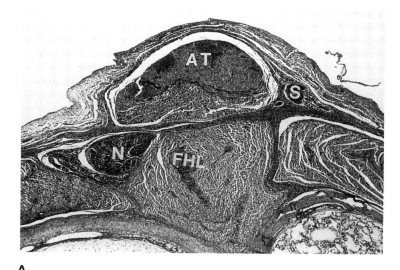

A

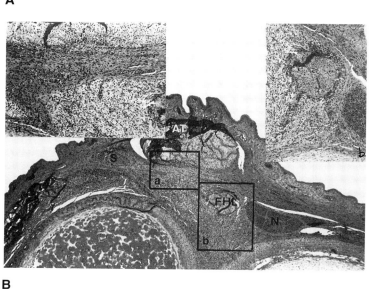

B

Figs 11A and 11B Transverse sections at the level of the distal tibial metaphyses of a 16-week-old fetus with a normal left foot (Fig. 11A Masson trichrone, × 90) and a right clubfoot (Fig. 11B, Masson trichrome, × 60). In the leg with the clubfoot, the fascia between the triceps surae and the deep muscles of the calf is greatly thickened and extends into the muscles, as illustrated in Inset **a** (× 180). At this level one sees only the tendo Achilles in the leg with the clubfoot, whereas there are abundant muscle fibers of the triceps surae visible in the normal leg. In the leg with the club foot, the superficial fascia is also thickened and merges with the subcutaneous tissue. In Inset **b** (× 120), one can see strands of fibrous tissue inside the flexor hallucis longus muscle. AT = tendo Achilles, FHL = flexor hallucis longus, N = posterior tibial nerve, S = sural nerve, Ti = Tibia, and Fi = fibula.

severe clubfeet that we examined in fetuses and neonates, the muscles of the anterior and posterior compartments of the leg were smaller in girth than in the controls. The muscle size correlated inversely with the severity of the deformity. With the light microscope, the muscle fibers, although somewhat small in circumference, appeared normal in all clubfeet, but the intercellular connective tissue was slightly increased. The proportion of muscle fibers to connective tissue was lowest in the triceps surae, tibialis posterior, and flexor digitorum communis. No appreciable differences were noted in the size of the peroneal muscles of the clubfeet as compared with the normal controls. Both the deep and the superficial fasciae of the calf were thicker in the clubfoot than in the controls. In the lower part of the leg, bundles of connective tissue fibers from the deep fasciae penetrated into the muscles. These abnormalities were of lesser degree in the moderate and mild clubfeet (Figs 11A, 11B, and 12).

Using histochemical techniques, some authors have described a predominant type 1 muscle fiber population in the posterior and medial muscle groups of clubfoot children (Isaacs *et al*. 1977; Mellerowicz *et al*. 1994). Electron microscope studies have shown atrophic angular fibers and loss of myofibrils. These findings suggest the presence of a regional neural abnormality (Handelsman and Badalamante 1981; Handelsman and Glasses 1994). Signs of neurogenic atrophy were observed in the abductor hallucis muscle in some clubfeet by Goldner and Fisk (1991).

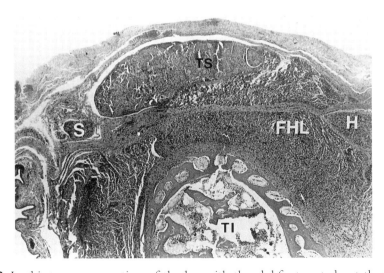

Fig. 12 In this transverse section of the leg with the clubfoot, cut about three millimeters above the section shown in Fig. 11B, there are more muscle fibers in the triceps surae and in the flexor hallucis longus than are seen at the level shown in Fig. 11B. The deep fascia is thick but sends fewer fibrous strands into the muscles (hematoxylin and eosin, × 150). TS = triceps surae, Ti = tibia, H = posterior tibial nerve, S = sural nerve, and FHL = flexor hallucis longus tendon within its muscle.

To study further the nature of the pathology in the leg muscles of clubfeet, I obtained muscle biopsies from the middle of the gastrocnemius of four patients with idiopathic clubfeet. These biopsies were obtained with two hemostats held separated and welded to a steel bar 1.5 cm long. Muscle biopsies were available from twenty age-matched controls. The patients were $1\frac{1}{2}$ to 10 years old at surgery for treatment of the deformity. In three patients the clubfoot was unilateral and in one bilateral. The patients had been treated by corrective manipulations and plaster casts during their first months of life. With Dr Maynard, we studied the muscles under the light and electron microscopes. Doctor Ionasescu investigated the *in vitro* collagen and non-collagen protein synthesis of the muscle ribosomes. Correlations between clinical, electron microscopy, and biochemical findings in the four patients are presented in Table 1.★

Specimens for light microscopy were fixed in formalin, embedded in paraffin and stained with Sirius Red, Mallory's trichrome, and hematoxylin and eosin. The sections revealed skeletal muscle free from excessive random variation in myofiber size. Endomesial connective tissue was increased in case 1, slightly increased in case 2, and normal in cases 3 and 4. There were no interstitial or perivascular inflammatory cell infiltrates. There were no central cores, nemaline bodies, or glycogen stores present.

For electron mycroscopy, the tissue was immersed in glutaraldehyde, embedded in Epon 812, sectioned and stained with uranyl acetate and lead citrate (Table 1).

Table 1 Correlations between clinical, EM, and biochemical findings

	Patient age (years)	Severity of deformity	EM collagen evaluation	*In vitro* protein synthesis of total polyribosomes	
				Collagen	Non-collagen
(1)	$1\frac{1}{2}$	R severe	increase	high	low
		L moderate	normal	high	high
(2)	5	L moderate	slight increase	high	slight increase
(3)	7	L mild	normal	normal	low
(4)	10	L severe	normal	normal	—

★ A patient I biopsied was included by error in the paper by Ionasescu *et al.* (1974). This patient was a three-year-old mentally retarded male with a moderate bilateral clubfoot deformity who exhibited in the gastrocnemius many myopathic changes such as myelin figures, loss of myofilaments, central nuclei, and spreading Z lines, in addition to extensive fibrosis. Degenerating muscle fibers were randomly scattered among normal fibers. This patient was the product of incest and had cerebral damage since birth and severe psychomotor dysfunction diagnosed after the biopsy. For these reasons, this patient is not included in this book since his clubfeet were not 'idiopathic'.

A considerable amount of intercellular connective tissue was evident in the right gastrocnemius of the $1\frac{1}{2}$-year-old patient, and there was a slight increase in the 5-year-old patient. (Fig. 13) Normal amounts of intercellular collagen were seen in the 7- and the 10-year-old patients.

The *in vitro* collagen synthesis of muscle polyribosomes was increased in the muscles of the $1\frac{1}{2}$-year-old and the 5-year-old patients, and it was normal in the two older ones. The non-collagen protein synthesis was decreased on the side of the severe right clubfoot of the $1\frac{1}{2}$-year-old patient; it was high in the moderate clubfoot of the same patient and only slightly increased in the 5-year-old patient. It was normal in the two older ones. [The procedure for the preparation of the muscle extracts and evaluation of ribosomal protein synthesis was reported by Ionasescu *et al.* (1970).]

The severity of the clubfoot deformity may be correlated with the pattern of protein synthesis in the gastrocnemius. This is well illustrated in the $1\frac{1}{2}$-year-old patient with bilateral clubfoot. Both collagen and non-collagen protein synthesis were high in the left gastrocnemius on the side of the moderate clubfoot,

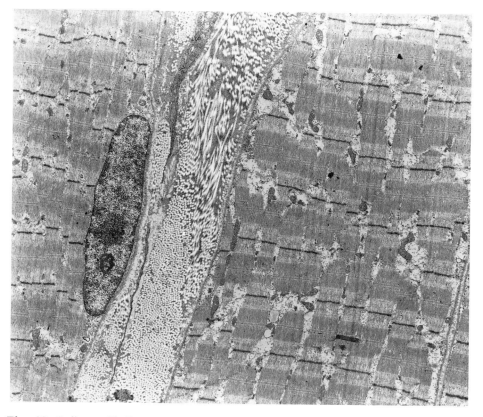

Fig. 13 Collagen fibrils are present in the gastrocnemius muscle of a $1\frac{1}{2}$-year-old baby with severe clubfoot (EM, × 6000).

whereas in the right gastrocnemius (the side with the severe clubfoot) collagen synthesis was high and non-collagen protein synthesis was low.

The normal amounts of intercellular collagen and the normal *in vitro* ribosomal collagen and non-collagen protein synthesis seen in the 7- and 10-year-old patients, correlates with the well-known clinical observation that the clubfoot deformity does not recur after 6 or 7 years of age.

Tendons

In fetuses and neonates, the distal part of the tibialis posterior tendon was increased two or three times in size and its sheath was thickened and matted to the ligaments in the medial aspect of the foot. Except for the tendo Achilles which inserted slightly medially on the posterior tuberosity of the calcaneus in one clubfoot, we did not find any anomalous tendon insertions in the fetuses and newborn babies we studied. However, in a 14-month-old child with unilateral clubfoot the anterior and posterior tibial tendons were united by a large tendon band lodged underneath the medial malleolus. Because of this very rare embryonic anomaly, the clubfoot deformity was corrected only after sectioning the tendon band. (Fig. 14) In a 6-month-old baby with rigid,

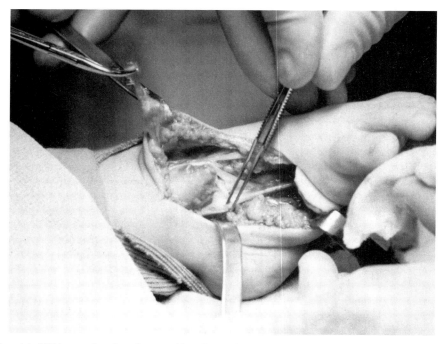

Fig. 14 Wide tendon band extending from the anterior to the posterior tibial tendon of a 14-month-old baby with clubfoot.

unyielding clubfeet the tibialis posterior tendon in the right foot inserted into the tuberosity of the navicular bone and gave off a very large fibrous expansion to the cuboid. The cuboid was displaced medially to the anterior tuberosity of the calcaneous in both feet, as observed in the roentgenograms taken at 3 months and at 6 months of age. The cuboid displacement was less severe in the left foot and improved after 3 months of manipulations whereas in the right foot the cuboid remained severely displaced. At surgery no abnormal tendon from the tibialis posterior inserted into the cuboid in the left foot (Figs 15A, 15B, 15C, and 15D).

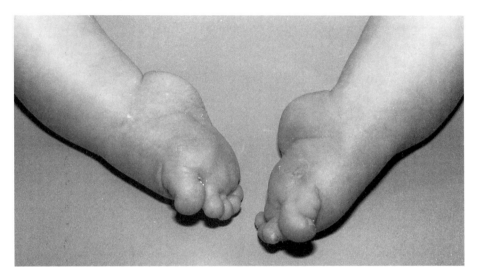

Fig. 15A Bilateral clubfeet of a 6-month-old baby resistant to manipulative reduction after the application of 10 plaster casts, started at 3 months of age.

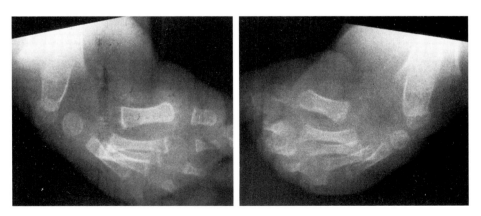

Fig. 15B Roentgenograms of the feet taken at 3 months of age. The cuboid is displaced medially to the anterior tuberosity of the calcaneous in both feet, more so in the right.

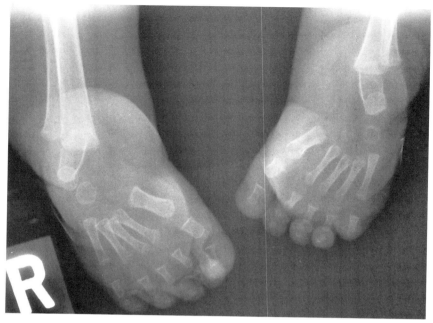

Fig. 15C Roentgenograms of the feet taken at 6 months of age. The alignment of the cuboid is improved in the left foot but not in the right.

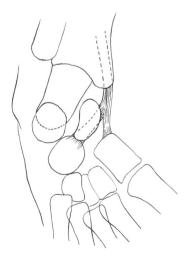

Fig. 15D Drawing showing a large branch of the tibialis posterior tendon inserting into the cuboid of the right foot. No abnormal tendon insertion was observed at surgery in the left foot.

In normal vertebrates, tendons are composed of long bundles of collagen fibers largely of type 1. The morphological and biochemical changes during maturation and aging in the Achilles tendon of the rabbit has been carefully studied by Ippolito, Cetta, Tenni, and other Italian researchers (Ippolito *et al.* 1980; Cetta *et al.* 1982). In the tendo Achilles of the New Zealand white rabbit, the collagen content increases with aging from 18 per cent (dry weight) in the late fetus (27 days *post coitus*) to 37 per cent in the newborn to 70 per cent in the 2-month-old to 85 per cent in the 4-year-old. The mean diameter of collagen fibrils increases with age, whereas the concentration of structural glycoproteins and galactosamine-containing glycosaminoglycans rapidly decreases. The same phenomenon has been described in the flexor tendons of the human hand during the very early stages of extrauterine life (Yuasa 1969).

The tendo Achilles of newborn rabbits has large amounts of spherical, elongated, or spindle-shaped cells called tenoblasts, arranged in long chains between the collagen fiber bundles. The cells have well-developed rough endoplasmic reticulum and Golgi apparatus indicating synthetic activity. Vesicles in the peripheral cytoplasm are associated with actin-like filaments. Unmyelinated nerves are found in contact with tenoblasts. The collagen bundles consist mainly of collagen fibers of about 370 angstroms in diameter. Some elastic fibers are seen adjacent to the tenocytes. Capillaries frequently run between cell chains.

In the 2-month-old rabbit, the cell-to-matrix ratio has decreased and all the tenoblasts are spindle-shaped and very elongated. The nucleus-to-cytoplasm ratio is increased. There is an increase in collagen matrix and in the number of large elastic fibers (Fig. 16).

In the tendo Achilles of the 4-year-old rabbit, the number of cells has decreased considerably. The diameter of the collagen bundles is greatly increased while the number of elastic fibers and capillaries have decreased. With specific antibodies, some actin and myosin were detected in the tendon cells at all ages by Ippolito *et al.* (1980) who observed that the size of the thin and thick filaments in the cytoplasm of the tenoblasts corresponded to the size of actin and myosin filaments. Other authors (Becker 1872; Handelsman and Badalamante 1981; Zimny *et al.* 1985) have demonstrated that actomyosin filaments in fibroblasts have morphological characteristics similar to those of smooth muscles. Ippolito *et al.* speculate that the contracting proteins in the tenoblasts may act on the elastic fibers, which are in close contact with the plasma membrane of the cells, thereby increasing the tone of the tendon and even strengthening a weak muscle contraction. Histologically, the structure of the tendo Achilles in children is similar to that of the rabbit.

While collagen in the rabbit tendon increases greatly in the first two months, thereafter it increases no more than 15 per cent. The number of elastic fibers markedly decreases with age. The same observations have been made in humans (Yuasa 1969). At all ages, however, elastic fibers are seen adjacent to the tenocytes. These contain actomyosin filaments. The presence of

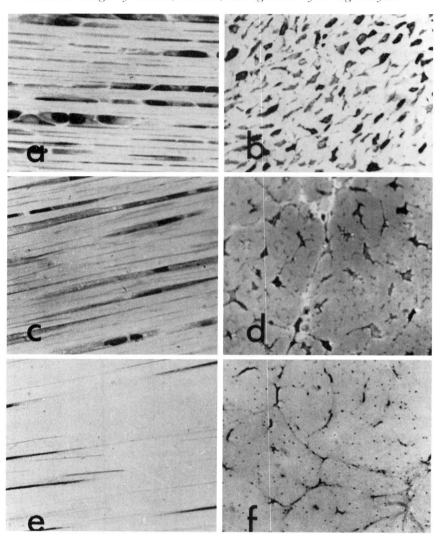

Fig. 16 Newborn rabbit tendon. (a) Longitudinal section showing tenoblasts of various shapes and sizes arranged in long parallel rows; (b) cross-section showing numerous cytoplasmic projections joining each other and surrounding first-order tendon bundles.

Young rabbit tendon. (c) Longitudinal section showing tenoblasts in decreased numbers in each row with a more uniform spindle shape; (d) cross-section showing that the cell-to-matrix ratio is decreased and the cytoplasmic projections are longer and more slender.

Old rabbit tendon. (e) Longitudinal section showing extremely elongaged tenoblasts with each cell mostly occupied by a long, thin nucleus: (f) cross-section showing that the cell-to-matrix ratio is further decreased and the cytoplasmic projections extend very far from the cellular body (toluidine blue, × 500). (From Ippolito *et al*. 1980, with the author's permission.)

unmyelinated nerves in close relationship with the tenoblasts may be important in the contraction and relaxation of the tendon. According to Ippolito *et. al.*, because of the great number of intertenocyte junctions, 'a few nerves could excite a whole tendon, the stimuli being transmitted through the cell projections' (Ippolito *et al.* 1980).

Tendons are viscoelastic materials. With immobilization the tendons lose a significant amount of water content, glycosaminoglycan concentration, and strength. With exercise, there is an increase in collagen fiber size, in strength, and in firmness (Tipton 1967, 1975; Gabbiani *et al.* 1973; Gelberman *et al.* 1988; Woo *et al.* 1980, 1981).

Kiplesund *et al.* (1983) with the light and electron microscopes observed no alternations in the structure of the collagen fibrils, fibroblasts, capillary endo-thelium, and peritendinous tissue elements in the tibialis posterior tendon of infants with congenital clubfoot.

Ligaments

In the normal foot the ligaments behave as viscoelastic fibrous connective tissue binding the bones and allowing the joints to be flexible yet stable. The function of the tarsal joints is specially influenced by the ligaments between and around the adjacent bones. The ligaments and joint capsules serve also as signal sources for reflex systems of the locomotor apparatus. 'It is clear that ligaments have mechanoreceptors participating in motor control' (Brand 1989, 1992). In the clubfoot the ligaments of the posterior and medial aspect of the ankle and tarsal joints are very thick and taut and firmly restrain the foot in equinus and the navicular and calcaneus in adduction and inversion.

All ligaments are formed by bundles of collagen fibrils displaying a wavy appearance under a microscope, known as 'crimp'. The 'crimp' disappears when stretching the ligament. Ninety per cent of the collagen is of type 1 and less than 10 per cent is of type 3. Ligaments contain actin and fibronectin in very small quantities. The ligaments in rat fetuses are very cellular; in the adult rat the fibroblasts are much less abundant. Elastic fibers appear in small numbers towards the end of fetal life. In humans, the plantar calcaneonavicular ligament contains abundant elastic fibers. Proteoglycans and glycoproteins constitute less than 1 per cent of the ligaments total dry weight (Frank *et al.* 1988).

Immobilization of joints causes a decrease in stiffness and strength of the ligaments as well as of the bone–ligament junction. This decrease is related to an increase in the synthesis and degradation of collagen and a decrease in glycos-aminoglycans (Akeson 1961; Akeson *et al.* 1977). Woo and associates (Woo *et al.* 1975, 1987) also noted a softening effect on ligament substance with immobiliza-tion. This and other studies have shown that immobilization substantially affects the periosteal type of insertion site owing to subperiosteal resorption of bone causing an increased avulsion failure in ligament insertions (Jack 1950; Laros *et al.* 1971; Woo *et al.* 1983).

Tipton (1975) observed that after endurance exercises in trained animals the ligaments had larger-diameter collagen fiber bundles and a higher collagen content.

In clubfeet of fetuses and neonates there is an increase of collagen fibers and cells in the ligaments of the distal tibiofibular joint, of the posterior and medial aspects of the tibiotalar, the subtalar, and the talocalcaneonavicular joints as well as in the posterior tibial tendon and its sheath (Ippolito and Ponseti 1980). The tibionavicular and calcaneonavicular ligaments and the posterior tibial tendon and its sheath form a large fribrotic mass of very cellular tissue with thick, irregularly oriented bundles of collagen fibers. Some of the cells are elongated such as fibroblasts and fibrocytes and others have spherical nuclei (Figs 17A and 17B). The interosseous talocalcaneal ligament, on the other hand, is composed of thin, loose strands of collagen fibers (Figs 18A and 18B). In an electron microscope study of clubfeet in children, Zimny *et al.* (1985). observed fibroblasts with cytoplasmic microfilaments, myofibroblasts-like cells, and mast cells in the ligaments of the medial side of the clubfoot. The myofibroblasts contain the contractile proteins actin and myosin. The stimulus for their contraction may come from the mast cells. Neither myofibroblasts nor mast cells were seen in the lateral side of the foot where fibroblasts with dilated rough endoplasmic reticulum and cytoplasmic microfilaments were present. Zimny *et al.* (1985) suggest that the fibroblastic contraction of the medial ligaments could be the cause of clubfoot. Fukuhara *et al.* (1994) observed densely packed collagen fibers and myofibroblast-like cells in the deltoid and spring ligaments of fetuses with severe clubfeet. The findings of both Zimny and Fukuhara corroborate our pathological findings and agree with our hypothesis that a retracting fibrosis is the primary etiological factor of the clubfoot deformity (Ippolito and Ponseti 1980).

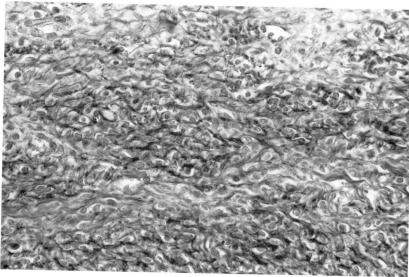

Fig. 17A Photomicrograph of the tibionavicular ligament of the right mild clubfoot in the 17-week-old fetus with bilateral clubfeet shown in Fig. 2. The collagen fibers are disrupted, fragmented, and densely packed. The cells are very abundant and many have spherical nuclei (Resorcinol–New Fuchsin van Giesen, × 475).

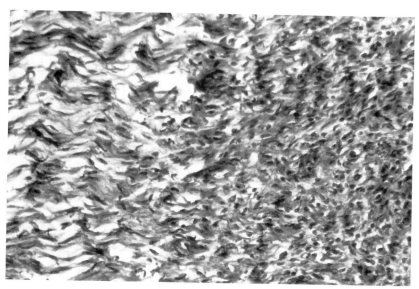

Fig. 17B Area of transition in the posterior tibial tendon. On the right the tendon is adjacent to the calcaneonavicular ligament and is very cellular and fibrotic. On the left we see the tendon branch to the second cuneiform with normal looking collagen fibers and a normal cell arrangement (Mason trichrome, × 718).

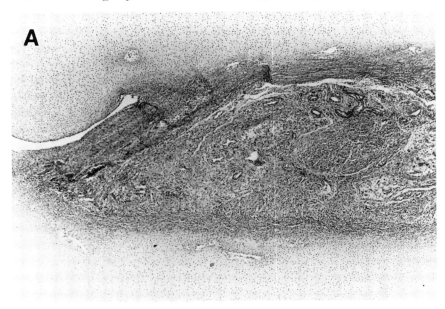

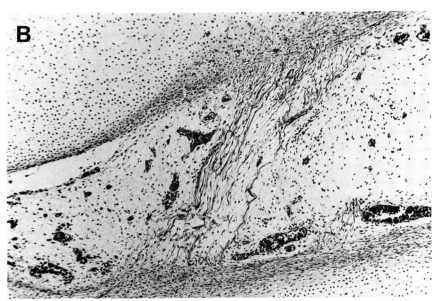

Figs 18A and 18B Sagittal section of the talocalcaneal interosseus ligament of a normal foot of a 20-week-old fetus (Fig. 18A, hematoxylin and eosin, × 200) and of a clubfoot of a 19-week-old fetus (Fig. 18B, hematoxylin and eosin, × 500). Unlike the normal foot, the ligament in the clubfoot is composed of thin, loose strands of collagen fibers.

References

Akeson, W.H. (1961). An experimental study of joint stiffness. *J. Bone Joint Surg.*, **43A**, 1022.

Akeson, W.H., Woo, SL-Y., Amiel, D., *et al.* (1977). Rapid recovery from contracture in rabbit hindlimb: A correlative biomechanical and biochemical study. *Clin. Orthop.*, **122**, 236.

Becker, C.G. (1972). Demonstration of actomyosim in mesangical cells of the renal glomerulus. *Am. J. Pathol.*, **66**, 97.

Brand, R.A. (1992). Autonomus informational stability in connective tissues. *Medical Hypotheses*, **37**, 107.

Brand, R.A. (1989). A neurosensory hypothesis of ligament function. *Medical Hypotheses*, **29**, 245.

Cetta, G., Tenni, R., Zanaboni, G., Deluca, G., Ippolito, E., De Martino, C., and Castellani, A. (1982). Biochemical and morphological modification in rabbit Achilles tendon during maturation and ageing. *Biochem. J.*, **204**, 61.

Frank, C., Woo, S., Andriacchi, T., Brand, R., Oakes, B., et al. (1988). Normal ligament: structure, function, and composition. In *Injury and repair of the musculoskeletal soft tissues*, (ed. S.L.-Y. Woo and J.A. Buckwalter, Chapter 2. American Academy of Orthopedic Surgeons, Park Ridge, IL.

Fukuhara, K., Schollmeier, G., and Uhthoff, H. (1994). The pathogenesis of clubfoot. A histomorphometric and immunobiochemical study of fetus. *J. Bone Joint Surg.*, **76B**, 450.

Gabbiani, G., Ryan, G.B., Lamelin, J.P., Vassalli, P., Majno, G., Bouvier, *et al.* (1973). Human smooth muscle autoantibody. *Am. J. Pathol.*, **72**, 473.

Gelberman, R., Goldberg, V., An, K-N., and Banes, A. (1988). Tendon. In *The injury and repair of the musculoskeletal soft tissues.* S.L.-Y Woo and J.A., Buckwalter Chapter 1. American Academy of Orthopedic Surgeons, Park Ridge, IL.

Goldner, J.L. and Fitch, R.D. (1991). Idiopathic congenital talipes equinovarus. In *Disorders of the foot and ankle*, 2nd edn), Vol. 1. (ed. M.H. Jahss), W.B. Saunders, Philadelphia.

Handelsman, J.E. and Badalamante, M.E. (1981). Neuromuscular studies in clubfoot. *J. Pediatr. Orthop.*, **1**, 23.

Handelsman, J.E. and Glasser, R. (1994). Muscle pathology in clubfoot and lower motor neuron lesions. In, *The clubfoot*, (ed. G.W. Simons), Chapter 1:21. Springer-Verlag, Berlin.

Ionasescu, V., Maynard, J.A., Ponseti, I.V., and Zellweger, H. (1974). The role of collagen in the pathogenesis of idiopathic clubfoot. Biochemical and electron microscopic correlations. *Helv. Paediat. Acta*, **29**, 305.

Ionasescu, V., Zellweger, H., Filer, L.L.J., and Conway, T.W. (1970). Increased collagen synthesis in arthrogryposis multiple congenita. *Arch. Neurol.*, **23**, 128.

Ippolito, E., Natali, P.G., Postacchinli, F., Accinori, L., and Martino, C.D. (1980). Morphological, immunochemical, and biochemical study of rabbit Achilles tendon at various ages. *J. Bone Joint Surg.*, **62A**, 583.

Ippolito, E. and Ponseti, I.V. (1980). Congenital clubfoot in the human fetus. *J. Bone Joint Surg.*, **62A**, 8.

Issacs, H., Handelsman, J.E., Badenhorst, M., and Pickering, A. (1977). The muscles in clubfoot: a histological histochemical and electron microscopic study. *J. Bone Joint Surg.*, **59B**, 465.

Jack, E.A. (1950). Experimental rupture of the medial collateral ligament of the knee. *J. Bone Joint Surg.*, **32B**, 396.

Kiplesund, K.M., Flood, P.R., and Sudmon, E. (1983). The ultra structure of tendon M. tibialis posterior in newborn infants suffering from congenital clubfoot. *Acta Orthop. Scand.*, **54**, 950.

Laros, G.S., Tipton, C.M., and Cooper, R.R. (1971). Influence of physical activity on ligament insertions in the knees of dogs. *J. Bone Joint Surg.*, **53A**, 275.

Mellerowicz, H., Sparmann, M., Eisenschenk, A., Dorfmuller-Kuchlin, S., and Gosztonyi, G. (1994). Morphometric study of muscles in congenital idiopathic clubfoot. In *The clubfoot*, (ed. G.W. Simons), Chapter 1:7. Springer-Verlag, Berlin.

Tipton, C.M., Schild, R.J., and Flatt, A.E. (1967). Measurement of ligamentous strength in rat knees. *J. Bone Joint Surg.*, **49A**, 63.

Tipton, C.M., Matthes, R.D., and Maynard, T.A. (1975). The influence of physical activity on ligaments and tendons. *Med. Sci. Sports*, **7**, 165.

Tipton, C., James, S., Mergner, W., and Tcheng, T-K. (1970). Influence of exercise on strength of medial collateral knee ligagments of dogs. *Am. J. Physiol.*, **218**, 894.

Woo, SL-Y., Gelberman, R.H., Cobb, N.G., Amiel, D., Lothringer, K., and Akeson, W.H. (1981). The importance of controlled passive mobilization on flexor tendon healing—A biomechanical study. *Acta Orthop. Scand.*, **52**, 615.

Woo, SL-Y., Gomez, M.A., Seguchi, Y., Endo, C.M., and Akeson, W.H. (1983). Measurement of mechanical properties of ligament substance from a bone–ligament–bone preparation. *J. Orthop. Res.*, **1**, 22.

Woo, SL-Y., Ritter, M.A., Amiel, D., *et al.* (1980). The biomechanical and biochemical properties of swine tendons—Long term effects of exercise on the digital extensors. *Connect Tissue Res.*, **7**, 177.

Woo, SL-Y., Gomez, M.D., Sites, T.J., Newton, P.O., Orlando, C.A., and Akeson, W.H. (1987). The biomechanical and morphological changes in the medial collateral ligament of the rabbit after immobilization and remobilization. *J. Bone Joint Surg.*, **69A**, 1200.

Woo, SL-Y., Matthews, J.V., Akeson, W.H., *et al.* (1975). Connective tissue response to immobility: Correlative study of biomechanical and biochemical measurements of normal and immobilized rabbit knees. *Arthritis Rheum.*, **18**, 257.

Yuasa, Y. (1969). Electron microscopic study on the development of the human fetal digital tendon. *J. Japanese Orthop. Assoc.*, **43**, 499.

Zimny, M.L., Willig, S.J., Roberts, J.M., and D'Ambrosia, R.D. (1985). An electron microscopic study of the fascia from the medial and lateral side of clubfoot. *Pediatr. Orthop.*, **5**, 577.

4
Functional anatomy

The kinematics of the tarsal joints in the normal foot have been studied for over a century but even today there is much controversy among experts about how they actually move. Some authors, among them Manter (1941), Hicks (1953), Elftman (1935, 1960), and Inman (1976), maintain that the subtalar joints move around a fixed rotation axis whereas others, including Farabeuf (1893), Fick (1904), Virchow (1899), Huson (1961), and Siegler *et al.* (1988) claim that there is no fixed axis of rotation for these joints.

The anatomy and kinesiology of the tarsus of the normal foot and of the clubfoot are lucidly described by Farabeuf in his book, *Precis de manual operatoire*, first published in 1872 (4th edn, 1893). (I have not seen his first edition, published in Paris in 1872 to ascertain whether it contains the same description.) In the fourth edition, Farabeuf clearly illustrates how in the normal foot the calcaneus moves under the talus by rotating around the inner fibers of the interosseous talocalcaneal ligament. Owing to the inclined contours of the talocalcaneal joint surfaces, as the calcaneus rotates under the talus, it adducts, flexes, and inverts. Farabeuf used the metaphor that it tacks, pitches, and rolls. As the foot goes into varus, the calcaneus adducts and inverts under the talus while the cuboid and the navicular adduct and invert in front of the calcaneus and the talar head, respectively. Farabeuf considered the displacement of the tarsal bones in a child's clubfoot to be the most extreme positions caused by the excessive pull of the tibialis posterior abetted by the gastrosoleus, tibialis anterior, long toe flexors, and plantar muscles. He states that the deformity of the talar neck is not 'a morphological caprice of nature' but results from the 'molding' caused by the posteriorly displaced and inverted navicular. Farabeuf illustrates how the ossification center of the talus responds to the abnormal pressures of the displaced navicular. He further states that the skeletal deformities in the infant are usually reversible. If not treated, the subluxations of the navicular and the cuboid present at birth worsen with the progresive displacement of these bones until a nearthrosis develops. Although these deformities may be corrected, he warns, the soft tissues have a 'deforming power' causing recurrences. In Farabeuf's time, infants rarely received early treatment and surgery was necessary to correct the deformity in the older child (Fig. 19).

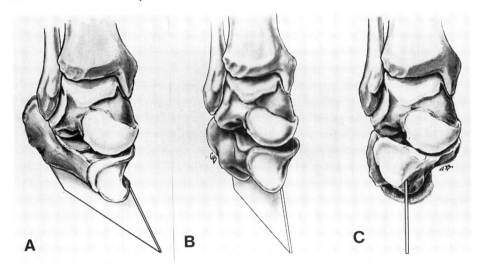

Fig. 19A In the clubfoot, the anterior portion of the calcaneus lies beneath the head of the talus. This position causes varus and equinus deformity of the heel. (B) Attempts to push the calcaneus into eversion without abducting it will not correct the heel varus. (C) Lateral displacement (abduction) of the anterior portion of the calcaneus to its normal relationship with the talus will correct the heel varus deformity of the clubfoot.

Huson's Ph.D. thesis in Dutch, 'A functional and anatomical study of the tarsus', published in Leiden in 1961, greatly advanced Farabeuf's observations and was a breakthrough in the understanding of the tarsal mechanism of the normal foot. His work revealed to me that my empirical observations on the kinematics of the clubfoot, made during the forties in the clinic, in the operating room, in dissected clubfoot specimens, and under cineradiography, were sound. Recently, Huson has published a chapter on the 'Functional anatomy of the foot' in Jahss's book, *Foot and ankle* (1991). Huson's followers, Van Langelaan (1983), and Benink (1985), have added important information on the kinematics of the tarsal joints and of the ankle in the normal foot. These works are basic for the understanding of foot kinematics.

Joint motions are determined by the curvature of the joint surfaces as well as by the orientation and structure of the binding ligaments. In the proximal part of the normal foot there is a complex combination of motions of the tarsal joints which are integrated in what Huson calls a 'closed kinematic chain' (*die kinetische kette*) (Payr 1927). The ligaments play an important role as 'kinematic constraints of the joints', apart from their share in forced transmission to support the elastic vault structure of the foot.

Huson demonstrated that the tarsal joints do not move as single hinges but rotate about moving axes as is the case in the knee. Each joint has its own specific motion pattern. Huson's work is supported by Van Langelaan, who, using a roentgenstereophotogrammetric method in post-mortem specimens, has shown 'that the motions of the tarsal joints can be described by means of a cone or fan-

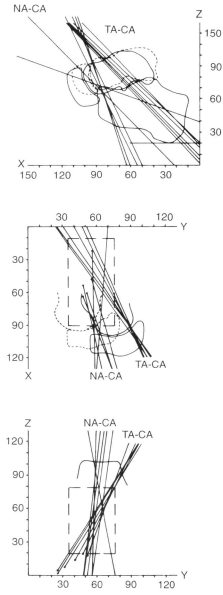

Fig. 20 Superpositioned axis bundles of the talocalcaneal (TA–CA) and calcaneo-navicular (NA–CA) joints. (From Van Langelaan 1983: A kinematical analysis of the tarsal joints. *Acta Orthop. Scand.* **54** (Suppl. 204): 1983.)

shaped bundle of discrete axes, representing the successive positions of a particular moving axis' (Fig. 20). He found that 'these successive positions followed fixed patterns which were characteristic for the joint concerned' and that 'according to these results, axes bundles could be established for all the tarsal joints'

(Van Langelaan 1983). Van Langelaan further observed that the magnitude of the total range of tarsal rotations varies from a mean of 23.6 degrees for the talocalcaneal joint, to a mean of 43.1 degrees for the talonavicular joint, and to only a mean of 15.8 degrees for the calcaneocuboid joint. The last two joints, therefore, have not only different axes bundles but also perform rotations of different magnitude (Figs 22I and 22J). Thus, as Huson summarizes, 'there is no such thing as a single Chopart joint, or midtarsal joint.' (Huson *et al.* 1986). Benink (1985) showed that continuous motions of the tarsal joints *in vivo* follow paths similar to the step-like motions recorded in Van Langellaan's experiments.

The calcaneocuboid joint has a 'close-packed position' when the loaded foot is in the neutral position. During inversion the surfaces of the calcaneocuboid joint are in restricted contact only and enter into a 'loose-pack position' regulated by the plantar calcaneocuboid ligament. The longest fibers of this ligament are located laterally and the shortest fibers are located on the medial side of the foot (Fig. 21).

The talocalcaneal joint also has its 'close-packed position' in the neutral position of the loaded foot and goes through 'loose-pack position' during

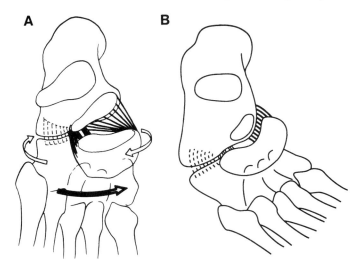

Fig. 21A Schematic dorsal view of the subtalar footplate of a normal foot demonstrating the arrangement of the longitudinally running plantar calcaneonavicular and calcaneocuboid ligaments. The shortest fibers are found in the midline of the foot whereas the longest are found at the outer margins of the foot. This arrangement allows inversion and eversion motions of the navicular and cuboid with respect to the talus and the calcaneus (*light arrows*) combined with an adduction of the navicular and cuboid (*heavy arrow*). (From Huson 1961.)

Fig. 21B In the clubfoot the shortening of the calcaneonavicular ligament and the medial displacement of the navicular greatly reduces the size of the subtalar foot plate and causes the foot to adduct in front and under the talus.

inversion, regulated by the strong strands of the deep talocalcaneal interosseous ligaments, which play a kinematic role similar to that of the plantar calca-neocuboid ligament (Figs 19A and 19C).

The talocalcaneonavicular joint is an arthrodial joint where the connection between the talus, the navicular, and the calcaneus is made (E.B. Smith 1896; J.W. Smith 1958). The plantar calcaneonavicular ligament forms part of the joint and supports the head of the talus while contributing to the maintenance of the arch of the foot (Fig. 21). This ligament contains abundant elastic fibers which contract during inversion (see Gray's *Anatomy*, 1973).

Motions of the tarsal joints occur simultaneously. If one of them is blocked the others are functionally blocked, too. This feature indicates that the tarsal joints belong to what Huson calls a 'constraint mechanism' (Figs 22I and 22J).

The ankle joint was well studied by Inman (1976). The axis of rotation of the ankle joint 'is not in the coronal plane but in one which passes from antero-medial to posterolateral'. In plantar flexion, the head of the talus swings in toward the medial side and the calcaneus inverts (Elftman 1935, 1960). The axis is not fixed but changes continuously throughout the range of movement. It may alter considerably during the arc of motion and differs significantly among individuals (Barnet and Namier 1952; Lundberg *et al.* 1989).

In the normal foot, rotations of the leg are converted by the tarsal mechan-ism into inversion and eversion motions of the foot. (Lundberg 1988, 1989). External rotation of the leg is followed by external rotation of the talus, causing the calcaneus to invert and abduct slightly owing to the slope of the posterior talocalcaneal joint. Inversion and slight abduction of the calcaneus cause inver-sion and adduction of the cuboid and the navicular, thereby raising the arch of the foot and thus inducing the first metatarsal to flex so that it reaches the ground. Inward rotation of the tibia causes the calcaneus to evert and the arch to flatten. In every one of these motions the ligaments are crucial structural ele-ments, especially the horizontally running fibers of the anterior talofibular liga-ment (Inman 1976; Huson *et al.* 1986). Benink extended Huson's work to living subjects and found that the input moment to be applied to the tibia to supinate the tarsus by rotation varied greatly from one individual to another (Huson *et al.* 1986). Benink (1985) described the tarsal index, determined by the relative positions of the talus and calcaneus in lateral roentgenograms. The tarsal indexes are low in cavus feet and high in flat feet.

There is no separation between the motion of the ankle and that of the subtalar joint in living subjects. Motion of the foot–shank complex in any direction occurs by the combined motions of both joints (called kinematic cou-pling by Siegler *et al.* 1988), and is the result of rotations at both the ankle and the subtalar joints. The contribution of the ankle joint to dorsiflexion/plantarflexion of the foot is larger than that of the subtalar joint. The con-tribution of the subtalar joint to inversion/eversion is larger than that of the ankle joint. 'The ankle and the subtalar joints participate about equally to internal/external rotation of the foot–shank complex' (Siegler *et al.* 1988).

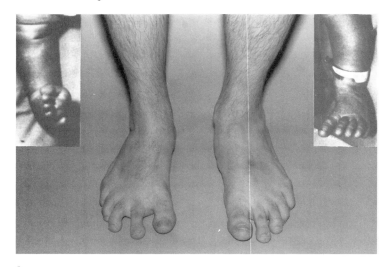

A

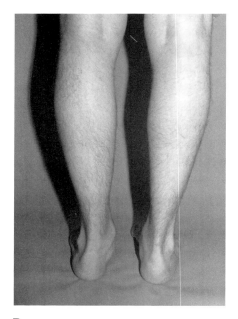

B

Figs 22A and 22B Front and back views of the feet of a 32 year-old male born with a right clubfoot and a left metatarsus adductus (*insets*). The clubfoot was treated with 5 plaster casts applied after manipulations. The casts were worn for a total of 7 weeks. The metatarsus adductus was treated with two plaster casts applied for a total of 4 weeks. The patient wore a foot-abduction bar at night for $2\frac{1}{2}$ years. The right shoe was fixed to the bar in a 60-degree external rotation; the left shoe was in the neutral position.

At 32 years of age, he is a construction worker on his feet the whole day without feeling any pain or discomfort. The right foot is $1\frac{1}{2}$ cms shorter than the left foot; the right leg is 2 cm shorter than the left leg; the circumference of the right calf is 2 cm smaller than that of the left calf. The right foot is well aligned; the left foot has a flat inner arch and the heel is in valgus.

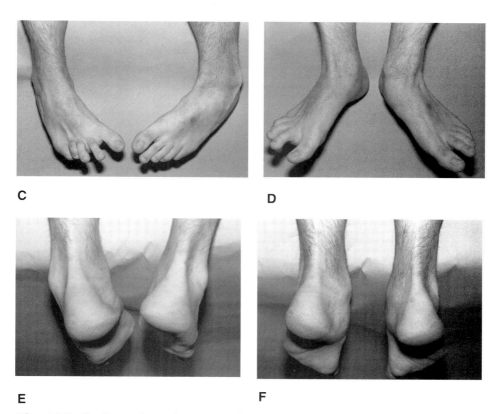

C

D

E

F

Figs 22C, D, E, and F The range of motion of the right hindfoot is restricted although the patient is not aware of this restriction. Motions of the forefoot are normal in both feet.

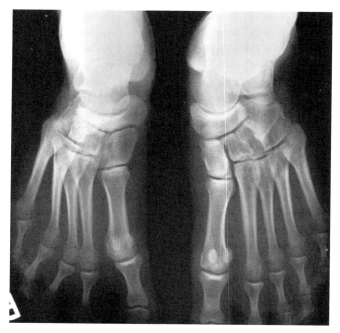

Figs 22G Standing roentgenograms of both feet. In the treated right clubfoot the navicular is wedge-shaped and flat and medially rotated as evidenced by the proximity of the tubercle to the medial malleolus. The talocalcaneal angle is 10 degrees in the right foot and 26 degrees in the left. The talar head is less spherical in the right foot than in the left one. In the right foot, the midfoot is in slight supinaton. The normal alignment of the right foot results, in part, from the lateral angulation of the cuneiforms and cuboid.

In the clubfoot, the kinematics are greatly altered by the severe shortening of the medial and posterior tarsal ligaments and by the tightness of the tibialis posterior and gastrosoleus muscles. The fibrotic and contracted deltoid ligament holds the calcaneus in inversion. The navicular is held severely medially displaced and inverted by the fibrosis of the tibionavicular, the plantar calcaneonavicular ligaments, and the pull of the tight tibialis posterior tendon (Attenborough 1966), (Fig. 21). In the sections of the fetuses studied, the talocalcaneal interossei, the bifurcate, and the naviculocuboid ligaments do not usually participate in the fibrosis. However, owing to the interdependence of the tarsal joints, the displacement of the navicular induces medial displacement and inversion of the cuboid and of the calcaneus. Invariably, the navicular and cuboid are severely medially displaced as well as inverted. The shape of the talar joint surfaces is changed, now adapting to the altered position of the tarsal elements (see Fig. 9 in Chapter 2).

The mobility of the posterior part of the foot is very restricted. In the severely supinated tarsus of a clubfoot, the range of passive motion varies

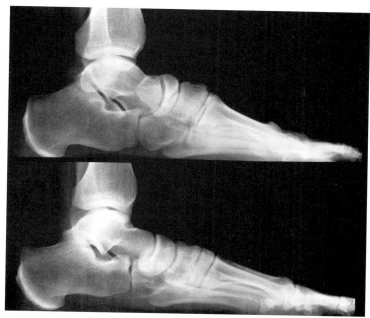

Fig. 22H Lateral standing roentgenograms. In the right foot (*above*), the sphericity of the talar dome is slightly dimished, the lateral tubercle of the talus is small, the sinus tarsi is large, and the navicular tubercle is close to the medial malleolus. The inner arch is of normal height in the right foot and flat in the left foot (*below*). All joints are of normal width in both feet.

greatly. Only a few degrees of passive abduction can be obtained in the tarsus of rigid feet, while 20 to 30 degrees are reached in less severe cases. Even with forced abduction, the tarsus of an untreated clubfoot cannot be moved to a neutral, normal position.

Although the tarsal bones are displaced and the tarsal joints are misshaped, they are congruent in the clubfoot position. In this position both the talo-navicular and the talocalcaneal joints are in a close-packed position. The de-formed surfaces of the calcaneocuboid joint are in restricted contact only. The joints become incongruent when correction of the deformity is attempted unless the correction is made gradually for several months allowing for the gradual remodeling of the joint surfaces. A surgical realignment of the skeletal elements requires severing most tarsal ligaments, causing all the tarsal joints to subluxate into a wholly unstable position.

The ligaments of the joints between the navicular and the cuneiforms, and those at the Lisfranc line and in the toes, are not involved in the fibrosis that affects mostly the hindfoot. Although adducted, the forefoot is less supinated than the hindfoot. Thus a cavus results with the first metatarsal in greater plantar flexion than the lateral metatarsals. The joints of the anterior part of the

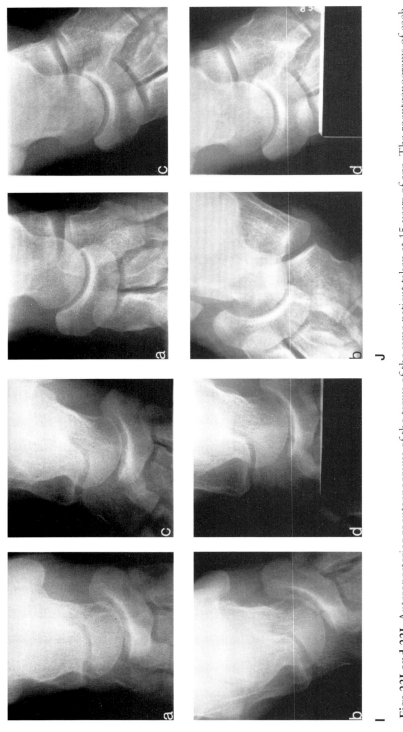

Figs 22I and 22J Anteroposterior roentgenograms of the tarsus of the same patient taken at 15 years of age. The roentgenograms of each foot were taken with the feet in different degrees of supination (**a** and **b**) and pronation (**c** and **d**). When the feet were supinated there was a wide range of tarsal shift in both feet owing to lax foot ligaments. The shift was greater in the navicular. There was some gapping in the calcaneonavicular joint. When the feet were pronated (**c** and **d**), however, there was some restriction of motion in the treated right clubfoot (Fig. 22 I).

foot are nearly normal even though the first cuneiformetatarsal joint may be medially slanted in some clubfeet, as observed in many feet with metatarsus adductus.

In the clubfoot, active and passive mobility of the anterior part of the foot and toes is only slightly restricted. In most cases at birth, the forefoot adduction can be corrected to a near normal position at the Lisfranc line, and the metatarsals can be flexed and extended through a normal range of motion. Even in cases where the first cuneiformetatarsal joint is medially slanted, the first metatarsal can be moved into the proper alignment with the other metatarsals, thereby eliminating the cavus.

The contrast between the stiffness of the severely supinated hindfoot and the suppleness of the forefoot poses a challenge to the orthopedist attempting to correct the deformity. The normal foot can freely supinate and pronate. However, attempts to pronate a clubfoot will only pronate the forefoot but not the hindfoot. Not only are the hindfoot ligaments very stiff, but the axes of motion of the tarsal joints are severely medially displaced resulting from the extreme medial rotation and displacement of the tarsal bones. Therefore, the hindfoot must be abducted in supination under the talus so that the tight medial ligaments can be stretched. The inversion of the calcaneus, navicular and cuboid will gradually decrease as the foot is further abducted (Figs 19, 22I, and 22J; see also Figs 32B and 32C, Chapter 7). Forceful pronation of a clubfoot will cause a breach in the midfoot and increase the cavus. We clearly observed this in the early fifties under cineradiography.

Most clubfeet cannot be completely anatomically corrected. After treatment there is some residual adduction of the tarsal bones as well as joint anomalies and some limitation of motion. In the severe clubfeet with very stiff medial tarsal ligaments a full reduction of the medial rotation of the navicular is not possible. The calcaneus cannot be fully abducted to its normal position under the talus. A partial correction of the tarsal displacements, however, is sufficient for a good function of the foot as illustrated in Fig. 22. The range of motion of the tarsal joints, although restricted, is compensated by the normal range of forefoot motion. Therefore, the range of motion of the whole foot is sufficient for the normal activities of living into the fourth decade, as attested by our last follow-up, and possibly for life. More detailed explanations will be provided in Chapter 7 when the treatment is discussed.

References

Attenborough, C.G. (1966). Severe congenital talipes equinovarus. *J. Bone Joint Surg.*, **48B**, 31.

Barnett, C.H. and Napier, J.R. (1952) The axis of rotation at the ankle joint in man. Its influence upon the form of the talus and the mobility of the fibula. *Anatomy*, **86**, 1.

Benink, R.J. (1985). The constraint mechanism of the human tarsus. *Acta Orthop. Scand.*, **56** (Suppl. 215).

Elftman, H. (1960). The transverse tarsal joint and its control. *Clin. Orthop.*, **16**, 41.

Elftman, H. and Manter, J. (1935). The evolution of the human foot with special reference to the joints. *J. Anat.*, **70**, 56.

Farabeuf, L.H. (1893). *Précis de manual operative* (4th edn). Masson, Paris. 1893. (First published 1872, Masson, Paris.)

Fick, R. (1904). *Handbuch der Anatomie und Mechanik der Gelenke.* Verlag G. Fischer, Jena.

Gray, H. (1973). *Anatomy of the human body*, 29th edn), (ed. C.M. Goss). Lea & Febiger, Philadelphia 1973.

Hicks, J.H. (1953). The mechanics of the foot. I. The joints. *J. Anat.*, **87**, 345.

Huson, A. (1961). Een ontleedkundig functioneel Onderzoek van de Voetwortel (An anatomical and functional study of the tarsus). Ph.D. dissertation, Leiden University.

Huson, A., Van Langelaan, E.J., and Spoor, C.W. (1986). The talocrural mechanism and tibiotalar delay. *Acta Morphol. Neerl.-Scand.*, **24**, 296.

Huson, A., Van Langelaan, E.J., and Spoor, C.W. (1986). Tibiotalar delay and tarsal gearing. *J. Anat.*, **149**, 244.

Inman, V.T. (1976). *The joints of the ankle*. Williams & Wilkins Baltimore.

Jahss, M.H. (1991). *Disorders of the foot and ankle*. W.B. Saunders, Philadelphia.

Lundberg, A., Svensson, O., Nemeth, G., and Selvik, G. (1989). The axis of rotation of the ankle joint. *J. Bone Joint Surg.*, **71B**, 94.

Lundberg, A. (1989). Kinematics of the ankle/foot complex. Part III: Influence of leg rotation. *Foot Ankle*, **9**, 304.

Lundberg, A. (1988). Patterns of motion of the ankle/foot complex. Ph.D. dissertation, Karolinska Institute, University of Stockholm.

Manter, J.B.T. (1941). Movements of the subtalar and transverse tarsal joints. *Anat. Rec.*, **80**, 397.

Payr, E. (1927). Der heutige stand der Gelenkchirurgie. *Archiv für Clin. Chir.*, **148**, 404.

Siegler, S., Cheu, J., and Schenck, C.D. (1988). Three dimensional kinematics and flexibility characteristics of the human ankle and subtalar joint. Part I: Kinematics. *J. Biomech. Eng.*, **110**, 364.

Smith, E.B. (1896). The astragalo-calcaneo-navicular joint. *J. Anat. Physiol.*, **30**, 390.

Smith, J.W. (1958). The ligamentous structures in the canalis and sinus tarsi. *J. Anat.*, **92**, 616.

Van Langelann, E.J. (1983). A kinematical analysis of the tarsal joints. *Acta Orthop. Scand.*, **54** (Suppl. 204).

Virchow, H. (1899) Über die Gelenke der Fusswurzel. *Arch. Anat. (Physiol. Abt.)* (Suppl), 556.

5
Pathogenesis

Very few cases of congenital clubfoot are due to environmental or extrinsic causes. Some authors feel that 'the clubfoot seen with congenital annular bands is secondary to the decreased capacity of the uterus resulting from early rupture of the amnion with the chorion remaining intact.' (Cowell and Wein 1980). Many clubfeet are a part of numerous syndromes in a strictly Mendelian pattern of either autosomal dominant or autosomal recessive inheritance (Wynne–Davies 1965). Also, cytogenic abnormalities produce individuals with syndromes including clubfoot, caused by excess cytogenetic material or by deletions of a portion of a chromosome. Many authors believe that the idiopathic clubfoot is primarily caused by a multifactorial inheritance system (Wynne-Davies 1965; Wynne-Davies *et al.* 1982). However, Rebbeck *et al.* (1993), using complex segregation analysis, favor the hypothesis that the deformity can be explained by the segregation of a single Mendelian gene plus other minor gene or non-genetic contributors (Wang *et al.* 1988).

Many theories have been proposed to explain the pathogenesis of the idiopathic clubfoot. Böhm (1929) and others have suggested that clubfoot results from an arrest of the development of the so-called clubfoot embryonic stage. Such a state, however, does not exist in normal embryos, and certainly the severe medial displacement of the navicular is not seen at any stage of the development of a normal embryo.

Some authors, including Waisbrod (1973), claim that there is a blastemal defect in the development of the tarsal cartilaginous anlage and that the soft-tissue changes are secondary to this defect. However, only one of the clubfeet studied by us, along with some clubfeet of young fetuses studied by others, showed minimal anomalies of the cartilaginous anlage. We did not find, in the anlage of the talus, the anomalies of the vascular channels described by Waisbrod to support this theory.

Other authors hold the hypothesis that the signals that provide positional information for the limbs with clubfoot are defective (Holland 1991; Tabin 1991). 'A complex interaction of morphogens, growth factors, and homeobox genes is probably necessary for informing cells and tissues of their proper location in the developing limb. A defect in this system might result in the malposition of tissues in clubfoot' (Rebbeck *et al.* 1993).

Severe bone deformities have been described in untreated idiopathic clubfeet of children and adults, and similar skeletal anomalies have been demonstrated in clubfeet of neurogenic origin, in which the anomalies presumably are related to a neuromuscular imbalance. The improvement in the skeletal deformities following manipulation and plaster cast treatment of many idiopathic clubfeet indicates the importance of properly directed mechanical stimuli in normal skeletal growth. The medial angulation of the neck of the talus observed in many clubfeet in fetuses and in early infancy was not seen in any of our treated patients in our 20- and 30-year follow-ups. All of these observations suggest that the abnormal positions of the cartilaginous anlage in the clubfoot of the fetus may be the cause of the skeletal deformities.

The congenital clubfoot deformity has been attributed to the abnormal tendon insertions observed by some authors. Except for a tendo Achilles which was inserted slightly medially on the posterior tuberosity of the calcaneus in one clubfoot, we did not find any anomalous tendon insertions in the fetus we examined. Whether the slightly abnormal insertion of the tendo Achilles in one foot was primary or secondary to the varus displacement of the heel is speculative.

Still other authors suggest that an abnormal position *in utero* or a small uterine cavity secondary to the loss of amniotic fluid may be the cause of the clubfoot deformity. Dietz states that 'evidence put forward for intrauterine moulding as a cause of idiopathic clubfoot does not stand up to scrutiny' (Dietz 1985). The presence in two of our specimens of a shortened triceps surae and of posterior ligaments pulled into the ankle joint suggests that the shortening of the muscle–tendon unit or other unknown factors may be primary and not secondary to an equinus position caused by external pressure. Further arguing against this theory is the fact that other conditions presumably caused by uterine pressure, such as calcaneovalgus and postural equinovarus feet, resolve spontaneously within weeks after birth.

Present-day sonography applied to the study of fetal development *in utero* has opened a new dimension in this field. Under sonography, we and others (Benacerraf and Frigoletto 1985; Jeanty *et al.* 1985; Bennacerraf 1986; Bronshtein and Zimmer 1989; Bronshtein *et al.* 1992 have observed that an apparently normal foot of an 11-week-old fetus turns into a clubfoot at 14 weeks within a uterine cavity filled with abundant amniotic fluid. The congenital clubfoot, therefore, seems to be a developmental anomaly originating in the third month of intrauterine life and not an embryonic malformation (Fig. 23).

Neuromuscular defects have been implicated in the causation of clubfeet. However, histological observations in the leg muscles of clubfeet in patients with neurological diseases are not relevant to idiopathic clubfoot. Similarly, clubfeet in patients with myopathies should not be mistaken for idiopathic. Histochemical and ultrastructural studies of leg muscles in patients with clubfoot have been reported recently. Some of these studies showed no abnormalities, whereas others showed changes suggesting regional neural anomalies such

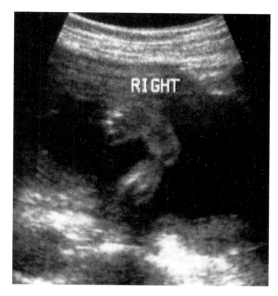

Fig. 23 Clubfoot of a 24-week-MA fetus seen with sonography. No clubfoot deformity was observed in this fetus with sonography at 12 weeks MA. At birth the baby had peripheral arthrogryposis as illustrated in the following Figure 24.

as an increase in type 1 muscle fibers (Isaacs *et al*. 1977; Handelsman and Glasser 1994). Increased fibrous tissue in the muscle–tendon junction of leg muscles has also been often observed. Therefore, the cause of the muscle imbalance presumably responsible for the deformity is not clear. Changes of neural origin in the leg muscles of idiopathic congenital clubfoot patients have not been unequivocably demonstrated either clinically or electromyographically.

Regardless of treatment, the circumference of the leg in all patients with unilateral clubfoot is smaller on the side with the clubfoot than on the normal side (Wiley 1959; Carrol 1990). Shortening of the muscle–tendon units in the leg, often associated with muscular fibrosis, has been frequently described in clubfoot (Wiley 1959). The bulk and the length of the calf muscles is diminished. In obese patients with unilateral clubfoot, the leg with the clubfoot has much less fat than the normal leg while the fat content in both thighs is about the same (see Fig. 51, Chapter 9).

Clubfeet tend to worsen and become more rigid soon after birth. The reason may be that there is a rapid synthesis of collagen in tendons and ligaments during the first weeks of life. This rapid collagen synthesis immediately preceding and following birth seems to be one cause of the great tendency of the clubfoot deformity to rapidly relapse after correction in premature babies and in early infancy. Collagen synthesis tapers down gradually until five or six years of age when collagen accretion in the ligaments is very low. Possibly, the intensive post-operative fibrosis and scarring observed after operative treatment in infants is related to the high collagen synthesis at this age. Less fibrosis occurs when surgery is delayed until 6 to 12 months of age (Green and Lloyd-Roberts 1985).

We found increased fibrous tissue in the muscles, fasciae, ligaments, and tendon sheaths of the posterior and medial aspects of the clubfoot specimens that we studied (Ionaseseu 1974; Ippolito and Ponseti 1980; also see Chapter 3, this volume). As mentioned earlier, in *An electron microscopic study of the fascia from the medial and lateral sides of clubfoot*, Zimny et al. (1985) have observed three cell types in fascia from the medial side of the clubfoot: typical fibroblasts, cells resembling myofibroblasts, and mast cells. Zimny *et al.* (1985) speculated that contracture of the medial tarsal ligaments in clubfoot may be due to the myofibroblast-like cells, and that this contracture may be enhanced by histamine released from the mast cells. Fukuhara *et al.* (1994) also observed myofibroblast-like cells in the spring ligament of clubfeet and speculated that the clubfoot deformity results from the fibromatosis in the medial tarsal ligaments, as Ippolito and I described in 1980.

Primary retracting fibrosis is seen in several disorders such as torticollis, idiopathic muscle fibrosis, and Dupuytren's contracture. Retracting scars are the most common example of connective–tissue contracture. We may speculate that genetically induced retraction of muscle–tendon units and of soft tissues in the leg related to a localized increase in collagen synthesis may be important factors in the causation of the clubfoot and its relapses.

Relapses occur within a few days in premature babies. Isaacs *et al.* (1977) suggested that minor innervation changes could be the prime factor in clubfoot development, and that muscle and tendon fibrosis could be a secondary change. Ionasescu *et al.* (1975) have demonstrated that there is a neurogenic control of muscle ribosomal protein synthesis.

Based on our present knowledge of clubfoot pathology and connective tissue biology, the clubfoot deformity seems to be induced by an unknown dysfunction in the territory subtended by the posterior tibial nerve below the knee. Some decrease in growth is found in the structures innervated by this nerve. Simultaneously, there is an excess of collagen synthesis with retracting fibrosis mainly in the tendo Achilles, the posterior tibial tendon, and the medial and posterior tarsal ligaments inducing the equinus and the medial displacement of the navicular, the heel varus, and the foot adduction.

The period of activity of any potentially abnormal 'neurotrophic factor,' presumably causing the deformity, varies. In severe cases, it may last from the tenth week of pregnancy to the sixth or seventh year of age. In mild cases, it may start in late fetal life and remain active for only a few months after birth. In all cases, the resulting fibrosis is most pronounced from a few weeks preceding birth to a few months after birth. This is the period, as we said earlier, when collagen accretion is greatest in tendons and ligaments of normal mammals and, presumably, also of man. Biochemical studies of the medial tarsal ligaments in fetuses and neonates may yield important information.

Regardless of cause, our observations on the pathogenesis of the deformity reported above are important for the proper treatment of clubfoot.

References

Benacerraf, B.R. (1986). Antenatal sonographic diagnosis of congenital clubfoot. A possible indication for amniocentesis. *J. Clin. Ultrasound*, **14**, 703.

Benacerraf, B.R. and Frigoletto, F.D. (1985). Prenatal ultrasound diagnosis of clubfoot. *Radiology*, **155**, 211.

Bohm, M. (1929). The embryologic origin of club-foot. *J. Bone Joint Surg.*, **11**, 229.

Bronshtein, M. and Zimmer, E.Z.: Transvaginal ultrasound diagnosis of fetal clubfeet at 13 weeks, menstrual age. *J. Clin. Ultrasound*, **17**, 518.

Bronshtein, M., Liberson, A., Lieberson, S., and Blumenfeld, Z. (1992). Clubfeet associated with hydrocephalus: new evidence of gradual dynamic development *in utero*. *Obstetrics and Gynecology*, **79**, 864.

Carroll, N. (1990). Clubfoot. In *Pediatric orthopaedics*, (3rd edn), (ed. R.T. Morrisy), J.P. Lippincott, Philadelphia.

Cowell, J.R. and Wein, B.K. (1980). Genetic aspects of clubfoot. *J. Bone Joint Surg.*, **62A**, 1381.

Dietz, F.R. (1985). On the pathogenesis of clubfoot. *Lancet*, **1**, 388.

Fukuhara, K., Schollmeier, G., and Uhthoff, H. (1994). The pathogenesis of clubfoot: A histomorphometric and immunhistochemical study of fetuses. *J. Bone Joint Surg.*, **76B**, 450.

Green, A.D.L. and Lloyd-Roberts, G.C. (1985). The results of early posterior release in resistant clubfeet. *J. Bone Joint Surg.*, **67B**, 588.

Handelsman, J.E. and Glasser, R. (1994). Muscle pathology in clubfoot and lower motor neuron lesions. In *The clubfoot*, (ed. G.W. Simons), Springer-Verlag, New York. 1994.

Holland, P.W. (1991). Cloning and evolutionary analysis of msh-like homeobox genes from mouse, zebrasfish, and ascidian. *Gene*, **98**, 253.

Ionasescu, V., Maynard, J.A., Ponseti, I.V., and Zellweger, H. (1974). The role of collagen in the pathogenesis of idiopathic clubfoot. Biochemical and electron microscopic correlations. *Helv. Paediatr. Acta*, **29**, 305.

Ionasescu, V., Lewis, R., and Schottelius, B. (1975). Neurogenic control of muscle ribosomal protein synthesis. *Acta Neurol. Scand.*, **51**, 253.

Ippolito, E. and Ponseti, I.V. (1980). Congenital clubfoot in the human fetus. A histological study. *J. Bone Joint Surg.*, **62A**, 8.

Isaacs, H., Handelsman, J.E., Badenhorst, M., and Pickering, A. (1977). The muscles in clubfoot: a histological, histochemical, and electron micrscopic study. *J. Bone Joint Surg.*, **59B**, 465.

Jeanty, P., Romero, R., d'Alton, M., Venus, I., and Hobbins, J.: (1985). *In utero* sonographic detection of hand and foot deformities. *J. Ultrasound Med.*, **4**, 595.

Kojima, A., Nakahara, H., Shimizu, N., Taga, I.; Ono, K., Nonaka, I., and Hiroshima, K. (1994). Histochemical studies in congenital clubfeet. In *The clubfoot*, (ed. G.W. Simons), Springer-Verlag, New York.

Rebbeck, T.R., Dietz, F.R., Murray, J.C., and Buetow, K.H. (1993). A single-gene explanation for the probability of having idiopathic talipes equinovarus. *Am. J. Hum. Genet.*, **53**, 1051.

Tabin, C.J. (1991). Retinoids, homeoboxes, and growth factors: toward molecular models of limb development. *Cell*, **66**, 199.

Waisbrod, H.: Congenital clubfoot: an anatomical study. *J. Bone Joint Surg.*, **55B**, 796.

Wang, J., Palmer, R., and Chung, C. (1988). The role of major gene in clubfoot. *Am. J. Hum. Genet.*, **42**, 772.

Wiley, A.M. (1959) An anatomical and experimental study of muscle growth. *J. Bone Joint Surg.*, **41B**, 821.

Wynne-Davies, R. (1965). Family studies and aetiology of clubfoot. *J. Med. Genet.*, **2**, 227.

Wynne-Davies, R., Littlejohn, A., and Gormley, J. (1982). Aetiology and inter-relationship of some common skeletal deformities. *J. Med. Genet.*, **19**, 321.

Zimmy, M.L., Willig, S.J., Roberts, J.M., and D'Ambrosia, R.D. (1985). An electron microscopic study of the fascia from medial and lateral sides of clubfoot. *J. Pediatr. Orthop.*, **5**, 577.

6
Clinical history and
examination

A family history and a general clinical examination of a baby with clubfoot should be obtained even after a check-up by a pediatrician. The family history should include a detailed inquiry into congenital defects of the locomotor system.

The baby should be fully undressed when inspected, first in the supine and then in the prone positions in order to detect possible anomalies in the head, neck, chest, trunk, and spine. A neurological examination should follow and the mobility of trunk and extremities should be evaluated.

The baby should be examined for possible anomalies in the range of motion of hips and knees. Stiffness or limitation of motion in joints other than the feet indicates bad prognosis because they often signify limited forms of arthrogryposis. Furthermore, short and very rigid clubfeet may be the only manifestation of peripheral arthrogryposis. The clubfeet in these patients are very rigid and difficult to correct. Surgical release of the tarsal joints and even talectomy are often needed (Fig. 24).

The length of the legs and the circumference of the thighs and calves should be measured. The skin creases in the thighs, the ankle, and the foot should be recorded as well as the degree of equinus, heel and forefoot adduction, cavus, and foot supination (Catteral 1991, 1994; Goldner and Fitch 1994).

Many degrees of severity and rigidity in the clubfoot components are found at birth. The orthopedist with trained fingers can easily determine the degree of displacement of the bones and the range of motion of the joints in the clubfoot. When examining the clubfoot it is advisable to keep in mind or in view a photograph of a well-dissected specimen (see Fig. 9, Chapter 2). The position of the malleoli in relation to the tibial crest and tuberosity, the head of the talus, and the calcaneal tuberosity should be noted. The degree of the following anomalies should be recorded: heel equinus, heel cord tightness, calf circumference and proximal retraction of the gastrosoleus muscle, adduction and inversion of the calcaneus, and the extent to which the talar head is subcutaneus in front of the lateral malleolus. The angle of forefoot adduction can best be measured from the sole of the foot (Alexander 1990). A severe metatarsus adductus must not be confused with clubfoot and treated as such. The result is a disastrous iatrogenic foot valgus deformity. The metatarsus adductus is easily differentiated from clubfoot because it has no equinus.

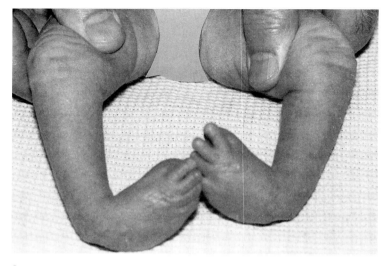

A

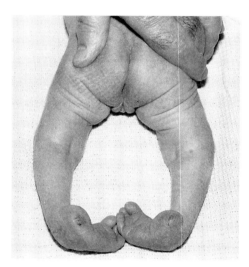

B

Figs 24A and 24B Severe, rigid clubfeet in the newborn baby girl with arthrogryposis confined to the legs. No muscle function was observed below the knees. The knees haa 20-degree flexion contracture.

To determine the position and range of motion of the navicular in the club-foot, the orthopedist should keep a steady grasp of the toes and metatarsals with one hand while he feels the malleoli from the front with the thumb and index finger of the other. The thumb should be on the fibular malleolus which is much more prominent than the tibial malleolus on which the index finger

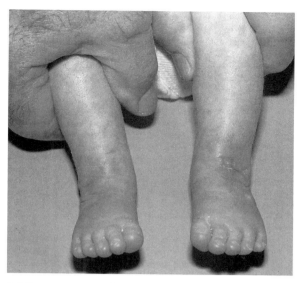

Fig. 24C The clubfeet were partially corrected with manipulations every 5 days and ten plaster-cast changes. A foot abduction bar could not be applied because both knees were laterally unstable and the thigh muscles were weak. A severe deformity recurred in spite of long leg braces. Early severe relapses are common in arthrogryposis. Joint release surgery or even talectomy are necessary.

rests. The tibial malleolus feels less prominent because the navicular abuts against its tip. As the the index finger and thumb slide down the malleoli, the thumb will come upon the prominent head of the talus while the index finger will reach the top of the navicular. With the hand holding the toes and metatarsals the foot is abducted while the index finger of the other hand pushes the navicular downwards and laterally. The distance between the medial malleolus and the navicular indicates the degree of displacement of the navicular. In the clubfoot the navicular tuberosity is in contact with the medial malleolus and resists separation. Only the lateral aspect of the talar head can be palpated with the thumb. In the normal foot the head of the talus can be felt between the index and the thumb in front of the medial and lateral malleoli (Figs 25 and 26).

It is easy to find by palpation the calcaneocuboid joint to determine the position of the cuboid and the degree of its displacement. Due to the looseness of the ligaments between the navicular and the cuboid, in most clubfeet the medial displacement of the cuboid will easily yield when the forefoot is abducted against counter pressure applied with the thumb on the lateral aspect of the head of the talus. The cuboid, however, may remain medially displaced when the orthopaedists apply counter pressure over the calcaneocuboid joint.

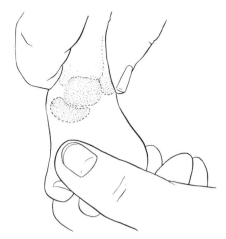

Fig. 25 The toes and metatarsals are grasped with one hand while the malleoli are felt from the front with the thumb and the index finger of the other hand.

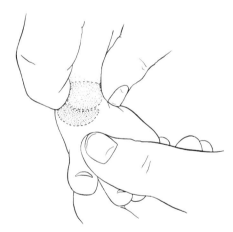

Fig. 26 The index finger and thumb slide downwards to reach the head of the talus and feel the navicular. With the hand holding the toes and metatarsals the foot is abducted and some motion is felt in the navicular. The distance between the medial malleolus and the navicular tuberosity indicates the degree of displacement of the navicular.

The cuneiforms can be palpated in front of the navicular. The first metatarsal is identified in plantar flexion. In most cases, it can be easily displaced in extension since the plantar fascia is usually not very tight if the infant has not been wrongly treated by immobilizing the forefoot in pronation.

The most important factors to be considered in determining the degree of severity of the clubfoot are: the reduction in size and degree of proximal retraction of the calf muscles; the severity of the equinus and varus of the heel; the rigidity of the adduction of the forefoot; the degree of medial displacement of the navicular; and the depth of the skin creases in the posterior aspect of the ankle and medial aspect of the foot. An experienced clinician can best judge the severity of the deformity after the first or second manipulations and plaster cast applications. The degree of lateral displacement of the navicular when abducting the foot is the orthopedist's main clue. Goldner and Fitch (1991, 1994) classify the severity of the clubfeet according to the distance between the navicular and the medial malleolus into severe (0–6 mm), moderate (7–12 mm), and mild (13–18 mm). In the normal foot their measured distance is from 19 to 24 mm (the same as measured by us in the roentgenograms of adults (see Chapter 10). Since Goldner and Fitch make no reference to the age of the patient, and the distance changes with age whether in a clubfoot or a normal foot, their figures should be taken with reservation.

An analysis of the anteroposterior and lateral roentgenograms of the foot may also assist the orthopedist in determining the extent of the deformities and in evaluating the treatment. However, it is difficult to estimate the accurate position of the tarsal bones in the roentgenograms of infants, because the centers of ossification of the three visible tarsal bones (calcaneus, talus, and cuboid) are small, oblong, and excentrically positioned. The navicular, the most displaced component of this deformity, does not ossify until the age of 3 or 4 years. I fully agree with Rose *et al.* (1985) who studied the flat foot in the child, that 'radiographs are not helpful, being flat images of a three-dimensional situation. Diagnostic lines and angles must be treated with great caution since they may show the same angle changed by viewing in a different axis. In addition, the ossific centers for all the foot bones do not appear until 4 years of age, and it is not until the age of 9 or 10 that features such as the sustentaculum tali can be seen. The axes of the foot bones can be drawn accurately only after the age of 6 years'. Cummings and colleagues (Watts 1991; Cummings *et al.* 1994) express similar concerns about the reliability of angle measurements of infants' feet. Furthermore, in our experience with long term results, the values of the talocalcaneal angles do not accurately predict the success or failure of treatment.

Unless the patient has been previously treated or has a very unusual deformity, I neither take roentgenograms of the infant's feet before nor after completion of the plaster cast treatment. In our hospital, treatment is usually started shortly after birth and the baby is only 2 months old or at most 3 months old at the end of the treatment, when splints are applied to maintain the correction. At this age, ossification is sketchy and the position of the head of the talus, navicular, cuboid, calcaneus, and forefoot can be best identified by palpation. The foot looks normal. Roentgenograms will be helpful if there is a relapse, which usually occurs after 1 or 2 years of age when ossification is more advanced.

References

Alexander, I.J. (1990). *The foot: examination and diagnosis*. Churchill Livingstone, New York, 1990.

Catteral, A. (1991). A method of assessment of the clubfoot deformity. *Clin. Orthop.*, **264**, 48.

Catteral, A. (1994). *Clinical assessment of clubfoot deformity*. In, *The clubfoot* (ed. G.W. Simons) Springer–Verlag, New York.

Cummings, R.J., Hay, R.M., McCluskey, W.P., Mazur, J.M., and Lovell, W.W. (1994). Can clubfeet be evaluated accurately and reproduciby? In *The clubfoot* (ed. G.W. Simons) Springer–Verlag, New York.

Goldner, J.D. and Fitch, R.D. (1991). Idiopathic congenital talipes equniovarus. In *Disorders of the foot and ankle*, (2nd edn), (ed. M.H. Jahss), Vol. 1. W.B. Saunders, Philadelphia.

Goldner, J.L. and Fitch, R.D. (1994). Classification and evaluation of congenital talipes equinovarus. In *The clubfoot*, (ed. G.W. Simons). Springer–Verlag, New York.

Rose, G.K., Welton, E.A., and Marshall, T. (1985). The diagnosis of flat foot in the child. *J. Bone Joint Surg.*, **67B**, 71.

Watts, H. (1991). Reproducibility of reading clubfoot x-rays. *Orthop. Trans.*, **15**, 105.

7

Treatment

The goal of treatment is to reduce or eliminate all the components of the congenital clubfoot deformity so that the patient has a functional, pain-free, normal-looking, plantigrade foot, with good mobility, without calluses, and requiring no modified shoes. A totally normal foot is not attainable and should not be expected.

We do not know the etiology of congenital clubfoot and we therefore cannot influence the pathology inherent in the ligaments, tendons, and muscles which seem to determine the degree of resistance to the correction and possibility of relapses.

Most orthopedists agree that the initial treatment of a clubfoot deformity should be non-operative and should begin in the first week of life in order to take advantage of the favorable viscoelastic properties of the connective tissue forming the ligaments, joint capsules, and tendons (Attlee 1868). Surgery in the clubfoot is invariably followed by deep scarring which appears to be particularly severe in infants. After extensive neonatal surgery, Dimeglio (1977) observed considerable fibrosis which 'progressively encased the foot in a fibrous block' (see also Epeldegui 1993). The abundant scar tissue forming after sectioning the joint capsules, ligaments, and muscles in clubfeet of infants may be related to the retracting fibrosis and to an increase of the collagen synthesis in these tissues, as we observed when studying *in vitro* protein synthesis in muscle biopsies from young clubfoot patients. The level of collagen synthesis appears to correlate with the degree of severity of the deformity (Ionasescu *et al.* 1974).

The abundant scar tissue formation after surgery is also related to the incongruent tarsal joint surfaces following capsular and ligament releases. As we said earlier, an immediate correction of the anatomic position of the displaced bones is impossible. The talonavicular, the talocalcaneal, and calcaneocuboid joint surfaces simply do not match after surgery. Indeed, wire fixation through the joint cartilage is needed to stabilize the bones in a roughly realigned position. Inevitably, the joint cartilage, as well as the joint capsules and ligaments, are damaged and joint stiffness sets in. The tarsal ligaments, like ligaments in any joint, are not expendable. They are indispensable in the kinematics of the foot. Furthermore, an exact anatomic alignment of the bones of the foot is not needed for a good functional result. For all these reasons, surgery is indicated only if a well-conducted manipulative treatment over a period of several months fails to correct the deformity, a rare occurence. In short, except for the rare, very severe, stiff clubfeet unyielding to manipulations, the results will be better if bone and joint surgery can be avoided altogether.

The manipulative treatment is based on the inherent properties of the connective tissue, cartilage, and bone, which respond to the proper mechanical stimuli created by the gradual reduction of the deformity. The ligaments, joint capsules, and tendons become stretched with gentle manipulations. A plaster cast is applied after each weekly session to retain the degree of correction and soften the ligaments. The displaced bones are thus gradually brought into the correct alignment with their joint surfaces progressively remodeled yet still congruent. Usually, after two months of manipulation and casting the foot appears slightly overcorrected. After a few weeks in splints the foot looks normal.

In some clubfeet, apparently tight ligaments seem to become easily stretchable under manipulation and the bones of the foot are easily aligned after the application of a few casts. In other clubfeet, the bone and joint deformities and the tight ligaments are more resistant to correction and require several more manipulative sessions and plaster cast applications. No more than ten plaster casts should be needed to obtain maximum correction. Further manipulations and immobilization may damage the osteoporotic bones rather than improve joint and bone alignment. Surgery is needed when the tight ligaments do not yield to the proper manipulations.

Without a thorough understanding of the anatomy and kinematics of the normal foot, and of the deviations of the tarsal bones in the clubfoot, the deformity is difficult to correct regardless of treatment, whether manipulative or surgical. Poorly conducted manipulations will further complicate the clubfoot deformity rather than correct it. Rough manipulations may tear the taut ligaments and cause scarring and stiffness, just as occurs after surgical intervention. The non-operative treatment will succeed better if it is started soon after birth and if the orthopaedist understands the nature of the deformity and possesses manipulative skill and expertise in plaster cast application.

Unfortunately, most orthopedists treating clubfeet act on the wrong assumption that the subtalar and Chopart joints have a fixed axis of rotation that goes from anteromediosuperior to posterolateroinferior passing through the sinus tarsi, and that by everting (pronating) the hindfoot on this axis the heel varus and foot supination will be corrected. This is not so. As explained in Chapter 4, there is no single axis (like a mitered hinge) upon which to rotate the tarsus in a normal or in a clubfoot (Huson 1991). What we have in each of the tarsal joints are oblique moving axes of rotation. In the clubfoot, these axes are greatly medially deflected owing to the extreme degree of medial displacement and inversion of the tarsal bones. Therefore, the correction of the severe tarsal misalignments necessitates a simultaneous, gradual lateral displacement of the navicular, the cuboid, and the calcaneus before these can be everted into a neutral position. The navicular must be brought downward from its nearly vertical position under the medial malleolus, laterally displaced, abducted, and finally, everted to a horizontal position to be properly aligned in front of the head of the talus. Simultaneously, the cuboid, although less displaced than the navicular, will have to be brought laterally and abducted before it is everted to its normal position in front of the calcaneus. At the same time, the calcaneus will need to be abducted in flexion under the talus before it can be everted to a neutral position. This is the procedure I have successfully used since 1948 on the basis of my anatomical and cineradiographic observations.

The poor results of the manipulative treatment of clubfeet in many clinics suggest that the attempts at correction have been inadequate because the techniques used are flawed. Textbooks and papers on pediatric orthopedics have devoted scant space to describing manipulative techniques in the treatment of this deformity and many of these descriptions, unfortunately, are faulty. The main errors are pronation of the forefoot and pronation of the whole foot shown as correct in illustrations (Figs 27A and 27B). Kite's (1964) book, *The clubfoot*, is atypical in that it describes his method in great detail and his method does not incur foot pronation. However, his technique is far from flawless. As mentioned in Chapter 1, he did not realize that the components of the clubfoot deformity are interdependent and must be corrected simultaneously to obtain good results. Consequently, his corrections, attained at great cost in time and effort, were not fully satisfactory.

After applying the plaster bandage to the foot, Kite set it 'on a glass plate to flatten the sole of the foot,' thereby correcting the cavus. Kite admonished not to 'push up and out on the forepart of the foot.' This way the cavus is prevented from recurring. He advises 'not to twist the foot out on the ankle,' thus avoiding foot pronation and a breach in the midfoot. He recommends, 'get all the correction by abducting the foot at the midtarsal joint' with his thumb pressing 'on the

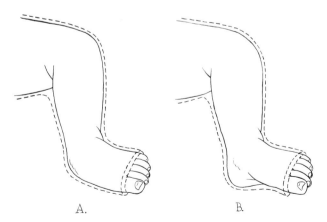

A.   B.

Figs 27A and 27B The main errors in the correction of the clubfoot are the pronation of the whole foot (A), and the pronation of the forefoot (B).

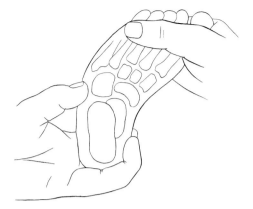

Fig. 28 (Kite's error). By abducting the forefoot against pressure at the calcaneocuboid joint the abduction of the calcaneous is blocked thereby interfering with the correction of the heel varus. Grasping the heel with the hand will prevent the calcaneus from abducting.

lateral side of the foot near the calcaneocuboid joint'. Unfortunately, by arching the foot against pressure at the calcaneocuboid joint 'as if one wanted to straighten a bent wire' (p. 119), he blocked the abduction of the calcaneus thereby interfering with the correction of the heel varus (Fig. 28). Kite wrongly believed that the heel varus would correct and 'his' talocalcaneal angle would open simply by everting the calcaneus. Therefore, it took a lot of patience and many months and cast changes to roll the calcaneus out from under the talus to correct the heel varus and obtain a plantigrade foot. Kite did not perceive that the heel varus is easily corrected by abducting the calcaneus under the talus so as to evert the calcaneus to a neutral position (see Fig. 19, Chapter 4). This flaw in Kite's technique has given rise to the disappointing results of his less patient followers who end up resorting to surgery (Kite 1930, 1963).

Although in our treatment all components of the clubfoot deformity except for the equinus are treated simultaneously, for greater clarity we will describe their correction separately: first the cavus, followed by the varus and the adductus, and lastly the equinus, which must be dealt with after the other components of the deformity are corrected. All manipulations should be very gentle. The deformity should be corrected slowly, and the ligaments should never be stretched beyond their natural amount of 'give'.

Cavus

The cavus or high arch is a very common component of the clubfoot deformity. The cavus is often confused with the forefoot equinus, also called plantaris, a rare deformity in which all five metatarsals are in nearly equal degree of plantar flexion. Occasionally, the plantaris is seen in a foot with congenital heel varus and adduction but without equinus. To correct the plantaris all metatarsals must be dorsiflexed simultaneously.

In most clubfeet the cavus deformity does not involve flexion of the entire forefoot. Rather, there is excessive plantar flexion primarily of the first metatarsal. Lateral roentgenograms of clubfeet often show the fifth metatarsal to be well aligned with the cuboid and the calcaneus, whereas the first metatarsal is in severe plantar flexion. Consequently, although the entire foot is supinated, the forefoot is pronated with respect to the hindfoot, thereby causing the cavus deformity (Fig. 29A). This deformity is, therefore, the result of the first metatarsal being in more plantar flexion than the last three metatarsals. In the normal foot as in the clubfoot, the forefoot can be twisted into inversion and eversion 'around a longitudinal axis formed by the second metatarsal solidly slotted into a socket formed by the cuneiform bones,' in Huson's (1991) words. A pronatory twist of the forefoot with a rise in the plantar arch occurs in stance in the normal foot when the leg externally rotates and the talus abducts forcing the calcaneus into inversion. In the clubfoot the arch can be very high.

Correction of the cavus component of the clubfoot is not addressed in most publications. In the 1940s, Steindler stated that 'the cavus deformity was one component which at times defied complete correction under the Kite treatment and, more often, under that of Denis Browne' (Steindler 1951). Certainly, the cavus can be improved with the Kite technique but not with the Denis Browne method of taping the feet on his L-shaped metal plates (Browne 1934). Even now, in many clinics, the cavus appears to be a difficult deformity

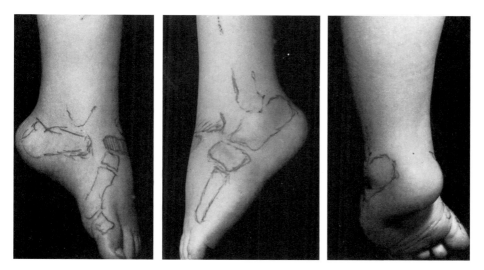

Fig. 29A Relapsed clubfoot of a 3-year-old boy. The foot is supinated, but the forefoot is pronated in relation with the heel. The first metatarsal is severely plantarflexed while the fifth is in proper alignment with the cuboid and calcaneus. This abnormal relationship between the forefoot and the hindfoot causes the cavus deformity.

to correct. Norris C. Carroll has stated that 'there is a cavus component to a severe clubfoot deformity' that 'can only be corrected by lengthening the plantar fascia and the intrinsic muscles' (Carroll 1987). Actually, the cavus can be easily corrected in most infants without surgery. Out of 104 clubfeet treated in our clinic and followed for over thirty years, only six feet needed plantar fasciotomy to correct completely the cavus (Laaveg and Ponseti 1980).

The plantar fascia and the abductor muscle are rarely very tight in the infant, and the fore part of the foot is usually flexible. Consequently, after gentle manipulation of the forefoot into supination and abduction, the cavus deformity usually corrects with the first plaster cast. While the cast is applied it is necessary to maintain the forefoot supinated and abducted in proper alignment with the hindfoot. The sole of the foot should be molded so as to maintain the height of a normal arch. By abducting the foot with counter-pressure applied on the head of the talus, not only is the adduction of the forefoot partially corrected by the first cast but, to a lesser degree, also the hindfoot adduction (Figs 29B and 29C). At this stage, since the whole foot is in supination, the inexperienced orthopedist may believe that the clubfoot deformity has been increased.

The first portion of the plaster cast should extend to the knee and maintain the whole foot in equinus, in supination, and in as much abduction as possible while mild counter pressure is applied over the lateral aspect of the head of the talus in front of the lateral malleolus. After the plaster sets, the cast must be extended to the upper third of the thigh with the knee flexed 90 degrees for reasons we shall explain later.

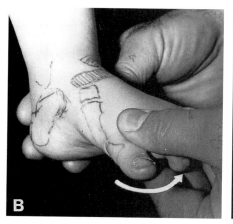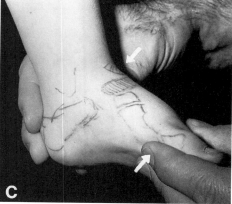

Figs 29B and 29C (B) Wrong maneuver to correct the clubfoot. The forefoot is pronated, and by plantarflexing the first metatarsal and dorsiflexing the fifth the cavus deformity increases and the heel varus does not correct. (C) The cavus is corrected by dorsiflexing the inner part of the forefoot, thereby placing it in proper alignment with the hindfoot.

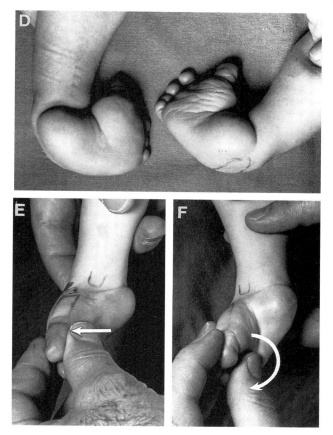

Fig. 29D Bilateral clubfoot deformity in a 6-week-old infant. The feet are severely supinated. The fore part of the foot is adducted and not as supinated as the hind part. The cavus deformity results from the slightly pronated position of the fore part of the foot in relation to the heel.

Fig. 29E Manipulation to correct the cavus deformity. The fore part of the foot is supinated so as to place it in proper alignment with the hind part of the foot.

Fig. 29F Wrong maneuver to correct foot supination. This maneuver increases the cavus deformity and fails to correct the varus deformity of the heel.

An attempt to correct the supination of the foot by forcibly pronating the forefoot increases the cavus deformity since the first metatarsal is further plantar-flexed (Fig. 29 B and F). Unfortunately, in most papers and textbooks, photographs show the forefoot held in pronation in the plaster cast. The cavus deformity remains uncorrected in this situation. In fact, it tends to increase and become more rigid when the forefoot is immobilized in pronation with respect to the hindfoot.

Varus and adduction

The varus and adduction as well as the equinus are the most severe deformities in a clubfoot and occur primarily in the hindfoot. The talus and calcaneus are generally deformed and in severe equinus, the calcaneus is in inversion and adduction, and the navicular as well as the cuboid are medially displaced and inverted. These components of the deformity, as mentioned earlier, are inextricably interrelated and usually are rigidly maintained by the shortened and thickened ligaments of the posterior aspect of the ankle and of the medial aspect of the foot and by the shortened muscles and tendons of the gastrocnemius, tibialis posterior, and toe flexors.

As explained in Chapter 4, the talocalcaneal, the talonavicular, and the calcaneocuboid joints operate in a strict mechanical interdependence. This is the reason it is necessary to simultaneously correct the tarsal displacements in the clubfoot.

The correction of the cavus brings the metatarsals, cuneiforms, navicular, and cuboid onto the same plane of supination. All these structures form the lever arm necessary to laterally and slightly downwardly displace the navicular and the cuboid. The lateral shift of the navicular, the cuboid, and the calcaneus in relation to the talus will be possible when the tight joint capsules, ligaments, and tendons on the inner aspect of the foot gradually yield to manipulation. This manipulation abducts the foot held in flexion and supination so as to accommodate the inversion of the tarsal bones while counter-pressure is applied with the thumb on the lateral aspect of the head of the talus. The heel should not be constrained so as to allow the abduction of the calcaneus under the talus. After two or three minutes of gentle manipulation, a thin, very well-molded plaster cast is applied over a thin layer of soft cotton. The tightness of the ligaments decreases with immobilization (Fig. 30A).

Three, four, or rarely five plaster casts changed weekly following gentle manipulations may be needed to loosen the medial ligamentous structures of the tarsus and partially mold the joints. In the first cast, the plantar flexed foot is in supination and in the following two or three casts the supination can be gradually decreased to correct the inversion of the tarsal bones while the foot is further abducted under the talus (Figs 30B and 30C). Care should be taken not to pronate the foot so as not to lock the calcaneus in varus under the talus. Care should also be taken not to evert the navicular while still in adduction. To ensure that the foot is not pronated, the plane of the sole and that of the metatarsal heads, which are in supination at the onset of treatment, should be gradually turned into a neutral position, so that they are at right angles to the leg in the last plaster cast when the inversion of the tarsal bones is fully corrected. The sole of the foot and the plane of the metatarsal heads should never be turned into pronation, to avoid an increase of the cavus and a breach in the midtarsal area (Fig. 29 and Figs 30B, 30C, 30D, and 30E).

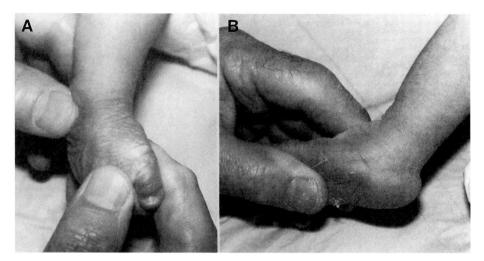

Figs 30A and 30B Manipulations to correct the cavus, varus, and adduction: outward presure is exerted on the metatarsals and counter pressure on the lateral aspect of the head of the talus. This manipulation abducts the foot held in flexion and supination. When the navicular, the cuboid, and the entire foot are displaced laterally in relation to the head of the talus, the anterior portion of the calcaneus follows; thus, the heel varus deformity is corrected.

Correction of the clubfoot deformity necessitates a prolonged stretching of the medial tarsal ligaments and tendons. This can be achieved only by external rotation of the whole foot under the talus to a much greater degree than is usually done by orthopedists (Figs 30E, 31A, and 31B). We must obtain 70 degrees of external rotation of the foot by the last cast after correction of the equinus (Figs 31C and 31D). This cast must be left on for three weeks. For several months thereafter, the foot must be maintained in 70 degrees of external rotation in shoes attached to a bar in order to prevent retraction of the medial tarsal ligaments (Fig. 34, p. 79).

In the normal foot the heel is in a straight line with the axis of the leg and 'eversion of the tarsal mechanism beyond its neutral position is very limited except for individuals with very relaxed ligaments (Huson 1961)' (Fig. 22, Chapter 4). Huson (1991) also states that 'starting from the neutral position the tarsal mechanism can perform only an inversion motion.' In the clubfoot, the severe varus of the tarsus is related to the severe adduction and inversion of its skeletal components. As stated earlier, correction of the heel varus entails abduction and external rotation of the foot distal to the talus. By this maneuver, the calcaneus will evert into its normal, neutral position. In most clubfeet, over-correction of the heel varus is neither possible nor desirable. In very severe cases, the distorted, laterally inclined posterior talocalcaneal joint can make correction of the heel varus difficult. The calcaneus in flexion will abduct

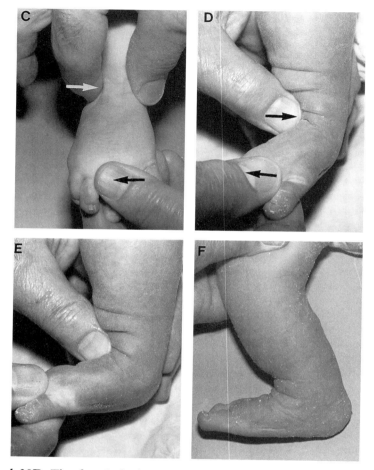

Figs 30C and 30D The foot is further abducted and the supination decreased but without pronating the foot.

Fig. 30E To stretch the middle tarsal ligaments the foot is abducted to 70 degrees. Note that the heel is not grasped by the hand thus allowing the calcaneus to abduct with the foot and the heel varus to correct.

Fig. 30F The equinus was corrected by subcutaneous section of the tendo Achilles and the foot was immobilized in a plaster cast for 3 weeks.

only gradually as the subtalar joint partially remodels. In less severe cases, owing to a more horizontal profile of the talocalcaneal joint surfaces and to the orientation of the tarsal ligaments, the inversion of the calcaneus often corrects itself when the foot is abducted under the talus even if the heel is not touched.

The foot can be maintained in external rotation only if the talus, the ankle, and the leg are stabilized by a toe-to-groin (to upper thigh) plaster cast while the knee is in 90-degree flexion. In order to maintain a strong external rotation of the foot under the talus while the talus is firmly immobilized against rotation in the ankle mortice, a toe-to-groin plaster cast is mandatory. The talar head will continue to stretch the tight plantar calcaneonavicular ligament as well as the tibionavicular part of the deltoid ligament, and the posterior tibial tendon just as we stretch them with manipulation. A cast extending to just below the knee cannot immoblize the foot in firm external rotation under the talus. The reason is that since the leg of a baby is round and the anterior crest of the tibia is covered with baby fat the cast cannot be well molded and therefore will rotate inwardly with the foot. As a result, the stretch of the tarsal ligaments and posterior tibial tendon obtained by manipulation is lost and the varus and ad-duction of the tarsus are left uncorrected. To insist on using short-leg casts in the treatment of clubfeet is to ignore the basic role that the leg and talus

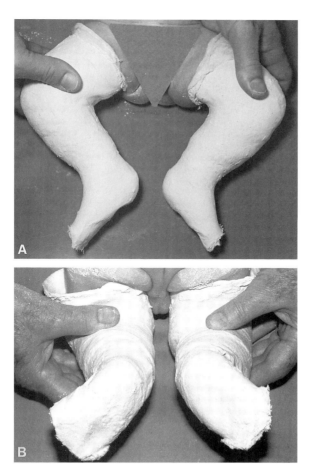

Figs 31A and 31B In the fifth plaster cast to correct the clubfoot of this baby the feet are abducted 50 degrees.

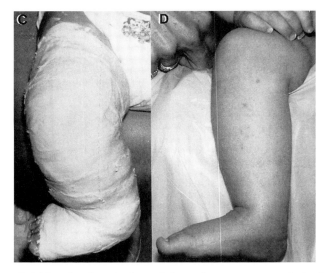

Figs 31C and 31D, In the sixth and last plaster cast applied after sectioning subcutaneously the tendo Achilles the right foot is abducted to 70 degrees (C) and not pronated. The foot is well corrected when the plaster cast is removed 3 weeks after surgery (D).

rotation have on the kinematics of the subtalar joint, the midfoot and the fore-foot (Inman 1976; Huson 1991). Furthermore, short-leg casts tend to slip off the foot. To prevent this, the orthopaedists often apply the casts too tightly around the calf and the malleoli, causing sores. Below-the-knee casts are not only useless but detrimental.

In severe clubfeet, complete reduction of the extreme medial displacement and inversion of the navicular may not be possible with manipulation, because the calcaneonavicular and the tibionavicular ligaments as well as the posterior tibial tendon, cannot be stretched sufficiently to properly position the navicular in front of the head of the talus. But even if the navicular were freed by cutting off the ligaments, the deformed contour of the talar head would be inadequate to accommodate it (see Fig. 9, Chapter 2). This is the rationale for stretching the medial ligaments as much as they will yield rather than cutting them, regardless of whether or not a perfect anatomical reduction is obtained.

With a partially reduced navicular, the forefoot can be brought into proper alignment with the hindfoot because the naviculocuneiform ligaments in front of the navicular, and the bifurcated ligaments yield and allow the lateral dis-placement and lateral angulation of the cuneiforms with respect to the navicular while the cuboid falls into normal position or in slight abduction with respect to the anterior tuberosity of the calcaneus. The calcaneus can be abducted sufficiently to bring the heel into its normal neutral position. This 'spurious' correction will provide good functional and cosmetic results and avoid the many complications of tarsal release surgeries (Figs 22 and 32).

The term 'spurious' is used here in the meliorative sense of 'superficially like but morphologically unlike' and not in the pejorative sense of 'false or fraudulent' (*Webster Tenth Collegiate Dictionary*). Orthopedists have accepted 'spurious' corrections of many skeletal deformities such as the correction of a coxa vara by an intertrochanteric osteotomy and not by an osteotomy of the femoral neck which could destroy the blood supply to the femoral head. For the same reason, the correction of a severe slipped upper femoral epiphysis is not done at the site of the growth plate where the slipping has occurred but by an osteotomy at a lower level. A third example of a 'spurious' correction is that of a severe tibia vara with an osteotomy at the upper tibial metaphysis and not through the upper tibial growth plate at the site of the disorder.

Relapses are common in severe cases of clubfoot for which a partial correction of the displaced navicular has been obtained. A bar with shoes holding the feet in 70 degrees of external rotation worn at night may delay or prevent a relapse. When a relapse occurs, transfer of the tibialis anterior tendon to the third cuneiform is needed. This treatment results in a nearly perfect clinical and functional foot for at least four decades. The treatment of relapses is addressed in Chapter 6.

Equinus

The equinus is corrected by dorsiflexing (extending) the foot with the heel in neutral position after the varus and adduction of the foot have been corrected.

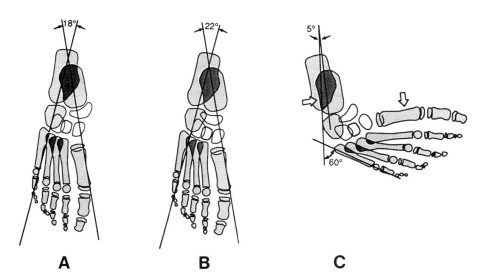

Figs 32A, 32B, and 32C Diagrams of the skeleton of a clubfoot (C) which is well corrected in (B). The medial displacement of the navicular and of the talocalcaneal angle are only partially corrected in (A).

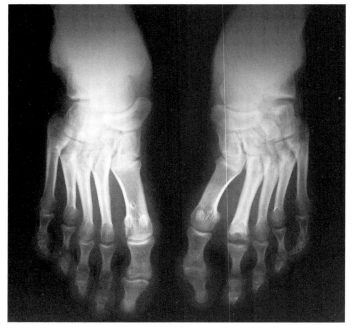

Fig. 32D Anteroposterior roentgenograms of a 19-year-old male born with congenital clubfeet. There is an incomplete correction of the medial displacement of the navicular and of the talocalcaneal angle in the right foot as depicted in the diagram in Fig. 32A. The left foot is well corrected; however, the talonavicular joint is narrow and the second metatarsal is dense and its head is flat. The feet were treated at 2 weeks of age with manipulation and plaster cast applications weekly until 3 months of age and with external rotation splints at night for 3 years. The tibialis anterior tendon was transferred to the third cuneiform at 8 years of age to treat a relapse. At this age the left foot had, in addition, a medial soft tissue release. The left foot is stiffer than the right and painful on long walks. (See Fig. 41.)

The correction of the equinus entails stretching the tight posterior capsules and ligaments of the ankle and subtalar joints and the tendo Achilles to allow the trochlea of the talus to slide backwards in the mortice. While the foot is extended, with one hand placed flat under the entire sole, the heel is grasped with the thumb and fingers of the other hand and pulled downwards. The index finger bent over the tendo Achilles insertion can also exert considerable pressure downwards.

Two or three plaster casts applied after manipulations, carefully molding the heel, are usually needed to correct the equinus deformity. Care should be taken not to cause a rocker-bottom deformity which can occur when the orthopedist attempts to dorsiflex the foot by applying pressure under the metatarsal heads rather than under the entire sole of the foot. When at least 15 degrees of ankle dorsiflexion, or more when possible, have been obtained, the last plaster cast is

applied and worn for three weeks with the foot in 70 degrees of external rotation. Special care should be taken never to pronate the foot in the slightest
degree so as to avoid a relapse of the cavus, a breach in the midfoot, and a
backward displacement of the lateral malleolus.

To facilitate the correction of the equinus when the tendon feels very tight
after the first manipulation to dorsiflex the ankle, a simple subcutaneus tenotomy of the tendo Achilles should be performed under local anesthesia to
obtain 15 degrees of ankle dorsiflexion. In this event, after the varus is corrected, one more plaster cast, worn for three weeks, will be sufficient to maintain the correction. Subcutaneus tenotomy is performed in about 85 per cent of
our patients for a faster correction. Dorsiflexion of the ankle to more than
10 to 15 degrees is often impossible because of the talar and calcaneal mal-
formations and tight ligaments. A posterior capsulotomy of the ankle and subtalar joints is rarely performed in our clinic because the additional degrees of
correction obtained by surgery may be completely lost later due to the retraction of the scar tissue. This is corroborated in recent reports from two leading
clinics. They indicate that posterior surgical release of the ankle in clubfeet is
followed by restriction of dorsiflexion and reduced mobility of the ankle in
nearly half of their patients (Hutchins *et al.* 1985; Aronson and Puskarich
1990).

Tibial torsion

Medial torsion deformities of the leg have been thought by some to be a component of the clubfoot deformity. However, in many treated clubfeet the lateral
malleolus is displaced backwards in spite of the alleged medial tibial torsion
(Hutchins *et al.* 1986). Several studies have attempted to determine the degree
of tibial torsion by measuring with a torsionmeter the angle between the bi-
condylar axis (or the tibial tubercle) and the bimalleolar axis. None of these
methods is accurate.

A new more precise method for measuring tibial torsion using computerized
tomography (CT) has been recently reported. It is solely dependent on tibial
landmarks and therefore measures true tibial torsion. The same technique is
applicable to ultrasound as well as to CT. Krishna *et al.* (1991) have measured
the angular differences between the proximal and distal posterior tibial planes as
defined by ultrasound scans in normal children and in children with clubfeet.
Normal children have a mean external tibial torsion of 40 degrees whereas children with clubfeet have a mean external tibial torsion of only 18 degrees. Of
interest is the finding that the normal legs of patients with unilateral clubfoot
have a mean external torsion of 27 degrees, considerably less than that of
normal children (Krishna *et al.* 1991).

Children with clubfeet, therefore, have no medial tibial torsion deformity
but rather half the amount of external tibial torsion than children with normal

feet. The posterior displacement of the distal fibula is caused by faulty treatment. Posterior displacement of the fibular malleolus and excessive lateral torsion of the ankle occurs when the foot is wrongly manipulated into abduction (external rotation) with the heel locked in inversion and adduction under the talus. Attempts to laterally rotate the foot in pronation with the heel inverted will force the talus to rotate laterally at the ankle joint, in turn displacing the fibular malleolus backwards. In addition, when walking with the heel uncorrected in varus and adduction, the child will turn his foot laterally to avoid tripping, causing further displacement of the fibular malleolus. A breach in the midfoot is incurred to make the foot plantigrade, causing a 'bean-shaped' deformity (Swann *et al.* 1969). This deformity is avoided when the heel varus is corrected by abducting and externally rotating the calcaneus under the talus with the foot in a neutral position. Placement of the thumb on the lateral aspect of the head of the talus helps prevent the talus from rotating laterally in the ankle joint.

The relative medial torsion associated with clubfoot will persist if below-the-knee casts are used in the treatment. Tibial torsion, varus deformity of the heel, and adduction of the foot can be gradually corrected if toe-to-groin plaster casts are applied with the knee in 90 degrees of flexion and the foot externally rotated under the talus, as we have described above. Splints with shoes in external rotation worn at night for many months will maintain the correction of the medial tibial torsion.

Plaster-cast application

The plaster cast is applied to maintain the correction obtained by manipulation. The baby often cries during manipulation and must be picked up from the table by the mother or the surgeon, patted and comforted, then placed at one end of the table to allow room for the assistant and the mother on either side, and relaxed with a bottle of warm milk or a pacifier. If the baby is breast-fed, he or she should be nursed before manipulation. The mother should remain close to the baby during all manipulative procedures.

During plaster cast application an assistant holds the thigh with one hand and the toes with the thumb and index finger of the other hand, maintaining the knee in 90 degrees of flexion. A 2-inch-wide rolled bandage of soft cotton is wrapped by the orthopedist overlapping by half the width, starting at the toes and proceeding upwards to the upper thigh. The reason for the overlapping is to cover the skin, including the heel, with just two thicknesses. Pressure sores are prevented not by overpadding but by careful molding. The soft cotton, as well as the plaster cast that follows, should be wrapped snugly over the foot and ankle for better molding and loosely over the calf and thigh to prevent unnecessary pressure on the muscles (Fig. 33A).

A two-inch plaster bandage, moistened in lukewarm water, is wrapped over the soft cotton starting at the toes; the toes should be covered by the tips of the

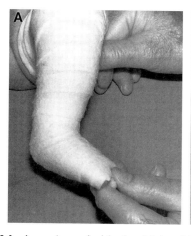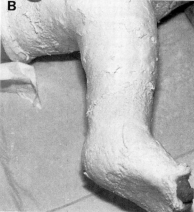

Fig. 33A An assistant holds the thigh with one hand and the toes with the thumb and index finger of the other hand maintaining the knee at 90 degrees of flexion. A 2-inch soft roll is wrapped from the toes to the upper thigh.

Fig. 33B In the second cast the foot is in some supination. The sole of the foot is well molded and the forefoot is not everted.

assistant's fingers to prevent crowding the toes. The plaster cast should extend to below the knee at first. Now, the assistant releases the toes as the surgeon takes hold of the foot to mold the plaster cast. Proper molding of the clubfoot necessitates a clear visualization of the position of each one of the bones in the foot. The surgeon should keep in mind an image of a dissected clubfoot (see Fig. 9, Chapter 2). The plaster cast must be molded with gentleness and anatomical precision.

The cast over the toes should be flattened to keep them in neutral alignment. The heel prominence should be emphasized by molding around it instead of pressing on it (Fig. 33C). The heel should never even rest on the surgeon's hand so as not to flatten it. A flat cast at the heel is a sure indication that it has been improperly applied.

When the foot is abducted to correct the adduction and supination, counter-pressure is applied with a thumb over the lateral aspect of the head of the talus. However, the thumb should never rest there for long, to avoid creating a dent on the plaster as it sets. The correction is maintained not through pressure but through molding. At the same time, the ankle and malleoli are gently molded. The heel should be molded in a neutral position taking care that it is not pushed into valgus. The heel varus corrects when abducting the foot. To help correct the equinus in the last casts, the heel is molded downwards with the bent index finger over the tendo Achilles.

After the foot and leg are molded and the cast is set, the leg should be supported by the surgeon's hand under the calf without ever touching the heel,

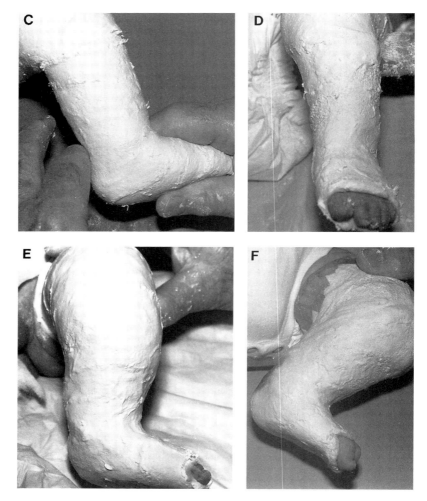

Fig. 33C The heel prominence is emphasized by molding around it instead of pressing on it.

Fig. 33D In the third plaster cast the foot is only slightly supinated and the adduction is corrected to a neutral position.

Fig. 33E In the fifth plaster cast the foot is markedly abducted without pronation.

Fig. 33F In the sixth plaster cast applied after subcutaneous section of the tendo Achilles the foot is held in 70 degrees of abduction and 25 degrees of dorsiflexion without pronation.

while the plaster cast is extended to the upper thigh, just below the groin, with the knee at 90 degrees of flexion and the leg in a slight external rotation (Figs 33E and 33F).

The plaster cast covering the toes should be trimmed to allow the toes to extend freely, but a platform of plaster should be left underneath the toes to prevent them from flexing. Otherwise, the tight toe flexors would remain unstretched. The plaster on the side of the big toe and the little toe should be trimmed away to allow the toes to move freely. The corrective force should be on the metatarsal heads, not on the toes.

In a newborn, the cast may be changed every four days for faster correction. However, after one month of age it is advisable to change the cast weekly. Six to ten toe-to-groin (to upper thigh) plaster casts, changed weekly except for the last cast which is worn for three weeks, should be sufficient to obtain correction.

Splinting

Following correction of the clubfoot deformity, splinting for many months is indispensable to help prevent relapses. Since the main corrective force of the varus and adduction of the clubfoot is abduction (that is, external rotation of the foot under the talus), a splint is needed to maintain the foot in the same degree of external rotation as it was in the last plaster cast. This is best accomplished with the feet in well-fitted, open-toed, high-top shoes attached in external rotation to a bar of about the length between the baby's shoulders. Since, unfortunately, commercial shoes for babies do not have a molded heel, a well-contoured strip of plastizote must be glued inside the counter of the shoe above the baby's heel to prevent the shoes from slipping off (Figs 34 and 35).

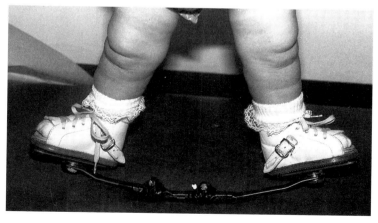

Fig. 34 External rotation splint. The shoes are fixed to the splint in 70 degrees of external rotation and in 15 degrees of dorsiflexion.

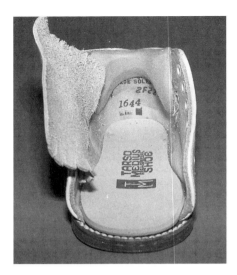

Fig. 35 A well-contoured strip of plastizode is glued inside the counter of the shoe above the baby's heel.

The splints are worn full time for two to three months and thereafter at night for two to four years. The splint should maintain the foot in 70 degrees of external rotation to prevent recurrence of the varus deformity of the heel, adduction of the foot, and in-toeing. The ankle should be in dorsiflexion, to prevent recurrence of the equinus. This is accomplished by bending the splint with the convexity of the bar distally directed. A splint or strapping that cannot firmly maintain the foot in marked external rotation without pronation is ineffectual. The added advantage of shoes attached to a bar as opposed to a fixed splint is that it allows motion of the feet, ankles, and knees. The baby may feel uncomfortable at first when it tries to alternately kick its legs. However, the baby soon learns to simultaneously kick both legs and the splints are well tolerated. In children with unilateral clubfoot the shoe for the normal foot is fixed on the bar in a neutral position.

The **L**-shaped plate advocated by Denis Browne (1934) for early correction of the clubfoot is ill-conceived since it attempts to correct the heel varus by everting without abducting the calcaneus, an impossible feat. First described in 1934, the concept of attaching the bandaged feet to plates held by a bar was not new. A device for the correction of clubfeet consisting of attaching to a bar contoured wooden platforms the size of the sole of the foot was proposed by Dr Henry Neil in 1825, described by John L. Attlee in 1868, and reported by L.A. Sayre in 1875 as explained by Le Noir (1966). The object was to have the child 'kick himself straight'. However, any such mechanical device cannot fully correct all the components of the clubfoot deformity. Only after the deformity is fully corrected is a bar attached to shoes in 70 degrees of external rotation effective in maintaining the correction.

No money should be wasted on any splint designed to prevent recurrence of the equinus which does not control rotation of the foot. Unless they are splinted in firm external rotation the pull of the retracting fibrosis in the ligaments of the medial aspect of the ankle and of the tibialis posterior and toe flexors is strong enough to cause a recurrence of the deformity in most feet.

Ordinary high-top shoes should be used for walking for two or three years, as they provide good stability for the ankle. Although outflare shoes and lateral wedges are recommended by many orthopedists, they are unnecessary if the foot has been corrected and ineffectual if the foot has not been corrected.

Surgery

When proper treatment of clubfeet with manipulation and plaster-casts has been started shortly after birth, a good clinical correction can be obtained in the majority of cases. The arbitrary classification of true clubfeet and positional clubfeet according to whether or not surgical correction has been effected is, as Coleman puts it, an 'artificial "preselection" concept' (Coleman 1987). If such classification were applied to our cases in Iowa, the number of true clubfeet vs. positional clubfeet would turn out to be 90 to 10 before 1950 (see Steindler 1951 and Le Noir 1966) and 10 to 90 after 1950, a ludicrous reversal.

An early surgical release operation may be indicated only in the small percentage (under 5 per cent) of patients who have short, unusually rigid feet with very severe equino-varus deformity, and who do not respond to proper manipulations. Such patients may be afflicted by peripheral artrogryposis and should be carefully studied. Recently, neo-natal clubfoot surgery and surgery in the first three months of life performed in leading clinics around the world has yielded very disappointing results owing to excessive deep scar formation (Dimeglio 1977; Epeldegui 1993). Most orthopedists have agreed that even in very rigid feet, surgery should be delayed until after the third month of life when post-surgical scarring is less abundant. Results from extensive dissections to release the stiff tarsal joints in infants are usually poor even after three months of age and further surgery at a later date is needed. During the first three months, therefore, attempts should be made to reduce the deformity as much as possible with manipulations and casting. Surprisingly, with a good technique, very difficult feet are often corrected.

After the removal of the last plaster cast, the orthopedist must clinically appraise the degree of correction obtained by manipulation. A foot with an acceptable correction will have the heel varus and equinus well corrected with about 15 degrees or more of ankle dorsiflexion. The navicular will be felt in front of the head of the talus, the cuboid will be well aligned with the calcaneus, and the shape of the foot will be normal. As previously explained, the position of the navicular is easily determined when it is felt moving in front of the head of the talus grasped with the index finger and thumb of one hand while adducting and abducting the foot with the other. In very severe clubfoot when the navicular cannot be fully laterally displaced, the navicular tuberosity is felt closer to the medial malleolus than in a normal foot (see Fig. 26, Chapter 6).

The degree of correction of the deformity can also be inferred from an analysis of anteroposterior and lateral roentgenograms of the foot. However, as stated before, it is difficult to estimate the accurate position of the tarsal bones because the centers of ossification are small, ovoid, and eccentrically positioned, and the navicular does not ossify until three or four years of age (Rose *et al.* 1985; Cummings *et al* 1994). It is important to understand that a talocalcaneal angle that is at some variance from the normal range does not signify a poor clinical result. Surgical release of the talar joints solely to obtain a normal talo-calcaneal index as viewed in roentgenograms is contraindicated. When the clinical correction of the foot and the motion of the foot and ankle are satisfactory, even though the correction may not be perfect on roentgenograms, the result of treatment should be considered successful.

In most clubfeet well treated by manipulations from early infancy, the only operations indicated to facilitate the treatment are tenotomy or lengthening of the tendo Achilles, and lateral transfer of the tendon of the tibialis anterior muscle to the third cuneiform. Joint releases should be avoided if possible since, in our experience, they cause stiffness, pain in adult life, and limited function.

Many techniques have been devised to release the tarsal joints in the treatment of clubfeet. No long-term functional results have been reported. The long-term follow-up on the Heyman–Herdon (Stark *et al.* 1987) tarsometatarsal capsulotomy for metatarsus adductus, published in 1987, showed that capsular release surgery on children's feet may cause severe disabilities. There was an overall failure rate of 41 per cent, an incidence of pain in 50 per cent, and degenerative changes in the operated joints. Surgeons should not ignore the consequences of joint damage inflicted by the extensive tarsal joint releases routinely performed in an effort to align the bones of a clubfoot deformity. The assumption that early 'correction' of bone positions results in a normal anatomy of the joints and good long-term function is a mistake.

A. Tendons

Tenotomy of the tendo Achilles

The percutaneous tenotomy of the tendo Achilles is an office procedure. An assistant holds the leg with the foot in dorsiflexion while the baby is relaxed with a bottle of milk. Under local anesthesia, a Beaver eye blade is introduced through the skin in the medial aspect of the tendo Achilles about two centimeters above its calcaneal insertion. The tendon is felt with the tip of the knife and care should be taken not to spear it. The knife is introduced in front of the tendon which is severed from front to back (Fig. 36). The angle of dorsiflexion of the ankle will suddenly increase some 10 to 15 degrees and the equinus deformity is corrected. The puncture wound is covered with a small sterile pad

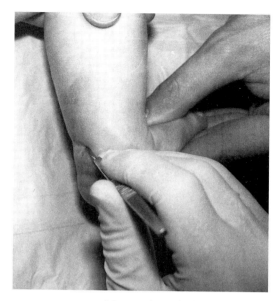

Fig. 36 Subcutaneous tenotomy of the tendo Achilles.

and a sterilized soft roll is wrapped around the foot, ankle, and leg, then a very well molded plaster cast is applied, maintaining the foot in maximum dorsiflexion and in about 70 degrees of external rotation, as described above. When the plaster cast is removed three weeks later, the space between the two ends of the tendon has been bridged. The scar left in the tendon is minimal, as observed in cases needing a tendo Achilles lengthening to correct a recurrence. During the first year of life a lengthening of the tendo Achilles through a skin incision is unnecessary.

Lengthening the tendo Achilles
Open lengthening of the tendo Achilles is indicated for children over one year of age. With the child under general anesthesia, a 2.5-cm-long skin incision is made over the medial aspect of the tendo Achilles about 3 cm above its distal insertion. The medial border of the tendon should be exposed by sharp dissection and the tendon sheath should be open longitudinally. The tendon should not be dissected from its sheath to avoid damage to the connective tissue strands that carry tiny blood vessels and nerve fibers from the sheath to the tendon. The tendon is split longitudinally in the frontal plane the length of 4 to 5 cm and severed posteriorly at the upper end of the incision and anteriorly at the lower end. The foot is dorsiflexed and the two halves of the tendon slide along each other and are sutured together with the ankle in 5 degrees of dorsiflexion. Excessive lengthening of the tendon must be avoided since it may permanently weaken the gastrosoleus. The tendon sheath is carefully closed before suturing the skin. The foot and leg are immobilized for four to five weeks in a long-leg plaster cast with the knee in slight flexion.

It is important not to make long incisions because they leave ugly scars. Long dissections of the sheath from the tendon leave large areas of the tendon devascularized. This may cause necrosis of the tendon with disastrous consequences. A 2.5-cm-long skin incision is sufficient to expose a long enough stretch of the tendon above and below the incision when flexing and extending the foot.

Transfer of the tibialis anterior tendon

The tendon is transferred after the first or second relapse in children older than two-and-a-half years of age when the tibialis anterior has a strong supinatory action. This often occurs when the navicular remains partially medially displaced and the varus of the calcaneus is not fully corrected. The relapsed clubfoot deformity must be well corrected with manipulations and two or three plaster casts left on for two weeks each before the transfer of the tendon. The tibialis anterior tendon transfer prevents further relapses and corrects the anteroposterior talocalcaneal angle as shown in the roentgenograms (Laaveg and Ponseti 1980). This transfer greatly reduces the need for medial release operations.

A 4- to 5-cm-long incision is made along the course of the tibialis anterior tendon from just below the ankle to the first cuneiform. The tendon sheath and the inferior extensor retinaculum are incised longitudinally and the tendon is severed just proximal to its insertion into the first cuneiform and first metatarsal. The distal end of the tendon is secured with a Kocher clamp and the tendon is lifted from its sheath up to its compartment under the superior retinaculum which is left intact. A second 2-cm-long incision is made over the dorsum of the foot centered over the third cuneiform. This bone is under the extensor digitorum brevis and is reached by retracting laterally the tendons of the extensor digitorum longus. The third cuneiform is identified by palpating its joint with the third metatarsal which is felt when extending and flexing the third metatarsal. A quarter-inch drill hole is made through the middle of the third cuneiform from the dorsal to the plantar aspects of the foot. The tendon of the tibialis anterior is passed subcutaneously to the second incision. The tip of the tendon is secured with two Keith needles and a Bunnell-type suture with a strong thread. With the needles the tendon is passed through the hole into the plantar aspect of the foot where it is firmly anchored over a piece of foam rubber and a button (Figs 37 and 38).

To prevent bow stringing of the tendon under the skin in front of the ankle, the tendon must be left under the superior retinaculum. To obtain a straight line of pull, the lateral septum of the retinacular compartment may be incised for a short distance. A toe-to-groin (to upper thigh) plaster cast is applied with the foot in neutral position and the knee at 90 degrees of flexion for four weeks (Figs 31 and 39).

B. Ligaments and joints

With appropriate early manipulations and plaster cast treatment of the clubfoot, surgery of the ligaments and joints should be rarely necessary. A very few

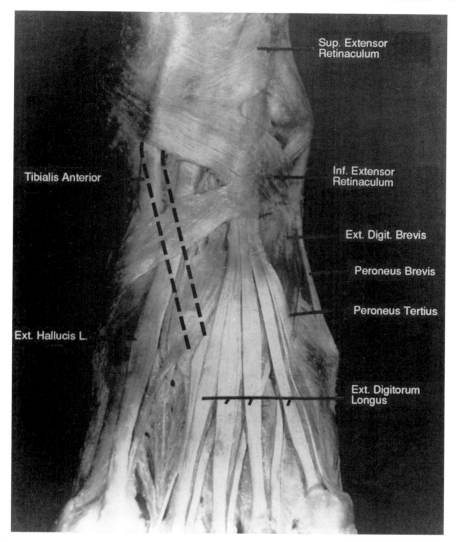

Fig. 37 Transfer of the tibialis anterior tendon to the third cuneiform. The tendon is left under the intact superior retinaculum (From R. Cosentino, 1960: *Atlas of anatomy and surgical approaches in orthopaedic surgery*. Charles C. Thomas, Springfield, IL.)

patients with severe deformities unyielding to manipulation treatment, in addition to patients with neglected clubfeet or with iatrogenic deformities, will be in need of joint releases. They should not be performed before five or six months of age. Maximum correction should be obtained with manipulative treatment and casting before undertaking any radical foot surgery.

Only the very tight ligaments should be sectioned to achieve a proper alignment of the bones, since a perfect anatomical reduction is unattainable owing

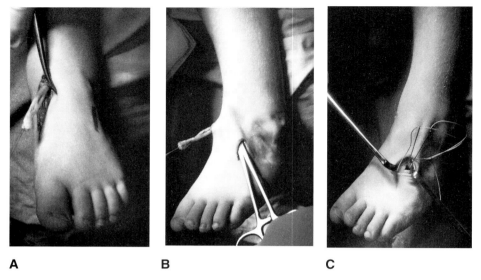

A   **B**   **C**

Fig. 38A, 38B, and 38C Transfer of the tibialis anterior tendon to the third cuneiform (see text).

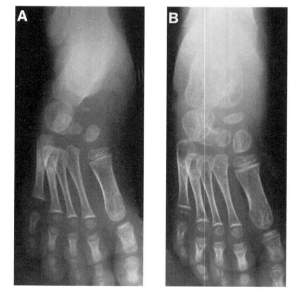

Fig. 39A and 39B Anteroposterior roentgenograms of a 4-year-old boy taken before (A) and 6 months after the tibialis anterior transfer to the third cuneiform (B). The talocalcaneal angle is improved.

to the incongruency of the joint surfaces and changes in the shape of the bones. As explained before, a complete reduction of the severe medial displacement of the navicular is not necessary for the correction of the heel varus and the medial angulation of the cuboid. If the foot is well aligned it is inadvisable to attempt to reduce completely the medially displaced navicular, since this requires an extensive dissection of the midfoot, sometimes with distressing results such as a navicular subluxation or dislocation and deep scarring. Le Noir (1966) as well as Simons (1994) describe severe medial subluxation of the cuboid that requires surgical reduction in some patients. Patients initially treated by me have not needed surgery to reduce the cuboid except in one instance when the clubfoot had a very large branch of the posterior tibial tendon that inserted into the cuboid.

The ligaments that may need to be released through a posteromedial incision are the superficial fibers of the deltoid ligament, the tibionavicular ligament, the talonavicular ligament, the plantar calcaneonavicular ligament, and the posterior ligaments of the ankle and subtalar joints (Fig. 40). Whenever the tibialis posterior tendon needs lengthening, it can be done following the technique described by Coleman (1987) of suturing the detached tendon to the flap of the tibionavicular ligament left attached to the navicular. Lengthening the tendons of the long toe flexors are rarely necessary since the muscles will stretch with time. The ligaments on the lateral aspect of the foot and the interosseous talocalcaneal ligaments are usually not excessively tight and should not be severed (Fig. 41). To avoid over-correction, the tendon of the tibialis anterior should not be transferred to the dorsum of the foot at the time of joint-release surgery.

Surgery to correct forefoot adduction should not be necessary since the forefoot is not rigid and easily yields to manipulation. A severe deformity may be corrected by metatarsal osteotomies but never by capsulotomies at the Listfranc line (Stark *et al.* 1987). Occasionally, a rigid cavus deformity will necessitate subcutaneous sectioning of the plantar fascia. A cock-up big toe can be corrected by transferring the long toe extensor to the neck of the first metatarsal as explained below.

C. Bones

Osteotomies or wedge resections of the bones on the outer aspect of the foot are not necessary in clubfoot treatment if manipulations and plaster cast applications are properly done.

Cavovarus

A common residual deformity of the poorly treated or of the relapsed clubfoot is the cavovarus, in which the tarsus remains in some degree of varus while the forefoot is pronated. The arch of the foot is high and the plantar fascia and muscles are shortened. This deformity usually originates from a faulty pronatory twist of the forefoot during the initial treatment. The cavus may be very mild at birth but it worsens when the forefoot is immobilized in pronation in a

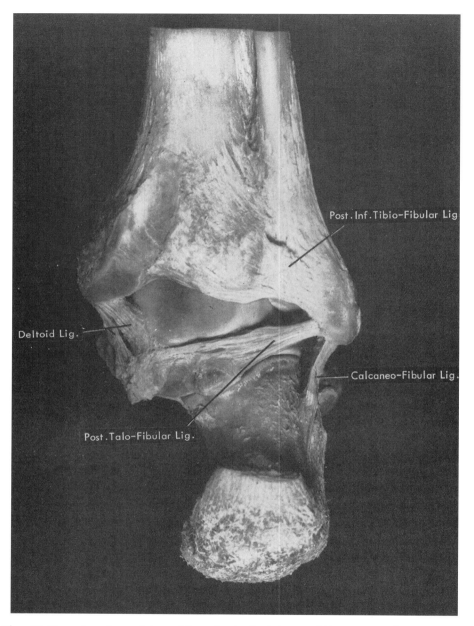

Post.Inf.Tibio-Fibular Lig

Deltoid Lig.

Calcaneo-Fibular Lig.

Post.Talo-Fibular Lig.

Fig. 40 Posterior view of the ankle and subtalar joints and ligaments to be severed at the posteromedial release operation. (From R. Cosentino, 1960: *Atlas of anatomy and surgical approaches in orthopaedic surgery*. Charles C. Thomas, Springfield, IL.)

plaster cast. Furthermore, the heel remains in varus since foot pronation cannot evert the calcaneus unless the midfoot and the calcaneus are severely abducted. With the heel in varus, the cavus increases when the child starts walking.

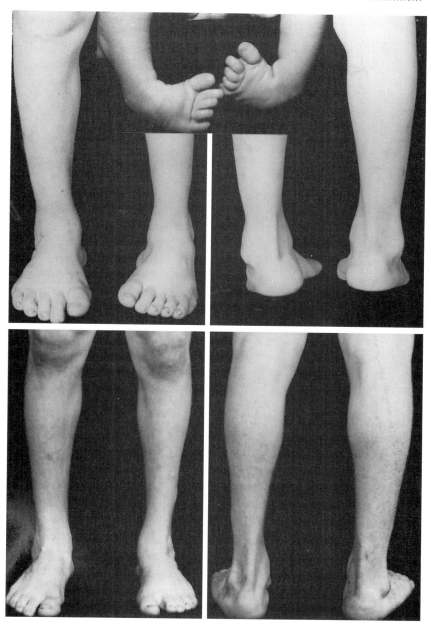

Fig. 41 Male with bilateral clubfoot, more severe on the left, treated as explained in the legend of Fig. 32D. The photos above show the feet before treatment and at 8 years of age when the deformity had relapsed. The photos below and the roentgenograms in Fig. 32D show the feet at 19 years of age. Both feet are well aligned. The left foot, treated with a posteromedial release operation, is stiffer than the right and painful on long walks. At 32 years of age, the patient had to give up farming because of increasing left foot pain. At 36 years of age, he drives maintenance trucks for the County.

The motions between the hindfoot and forefoot take place mainly at the Lisfranc line. The base of the second metatarsal is wedged between the first and third cuneiforms and therefore tends to move with the mid-and hindfoot. The forefoot twists into pronation and supination around the second metatarsal. In the cavovarus foot the hindfoot varus causes the second metatarsal to invert. When standing and walking, the first metatarsal has to plantarflex to reach the ground, while the lateral metatarsals have to dorsiflex. The plantar fascia becomes thicker and shorter as it holds the first metatarsal in plantar flexion. If there is a residual adduction of the foot, the child will walk with the leg in external rotation to avoid tripping, thus forcing the talus to follow in the same direction, in turn increasing the heel varus. The powerful anterior talofibular ligament plays an important role in what Huson calls 'this remarkable mechanism of talocrural transmission' (Huson 1991). All these interrelated motions create a vicious circle which keeps aggravating the condition.

The correction of the cavovarus deformity in clubfoot entails severing the plantar fascia and correcting the flexion of the first metatarsal and the supination of the tarsus. Steindler, who in 1920 published his plantar fascia release operation, stated repeatedly that the cavus would recur unless the plantar release was accompanied by some other corrective procedure.

The cavovarus residual deformity in children under six or seven years of age, when the subtalar joint motion is adequate, can be treated by manipulation, application of two or three plaster casts for two weeks each, percutaneous section of the plantar fascia, and transfer of the tendon of the tibialis anterior to the third cuneiform. The tendo Achilles may have to be lengthened when there is residual equinus. In severe cavus deformities, the extensor hallucis longus can be transferred to the shaft of the first metatarsal after attaching the distal end of the tendon to the tendon of the extensor hallucis brevis. A toe-to-groin plaster cast is applied holding the foot in the corrected position for five weeks.

In older children the tarsal deformity as well as the cavus tend to become more rigid. It is very important to find out with the Coleman's (1987) lateral block test whether the heel supination is correctable. Here a block of wood two or three centimeters high is placed under the lateral aspect of the sole of the foot so that the head of the first metatarsal touches the ground accomodating the forefoot pronation. If the hindfoot varus is not rigid, it will correct and the heel will no longer be in varus. When the heel varus corrects to within 5 degrees of the neutral position with the Coleman's test, the cavovarus deformity is best corrected by a series of procedures advocated by Reginald R. Cooper, as follows:

1. The tight plantar fascia is severed percutaneously.
2. A small dorsal–lateral wedge of bone is resected from the base of the first metatarsal, with care not to damage the growth plate.
3. The tendon of the extensor hallucis longus is severed at the level of the MP joint, its distal end is sutured to the tendon of the extensor hallucis brevis,

and its proximal end is passed through a drill hole in the shaft of the first metatarsal and tied to itself with a strong tension to hold the first metatarsal in proper alignment after it has been dorsiflexed and supinated (inverted) while immobilizing the osteotomy site.

4. Through a small lateral incision, the tendon of the peroneus longus is severed in the plantar aspect of the foot and sutured under tension to the tendon of the peroneus brevis.

5. The tibialis anterior tendon is transferred to the third cuneiform if it has a strong supinatory action.

6. The Achilles tendon is lengthened when necessary to correct any residual equinus.

7. A toe-to-groin plaster cast is applied holding the knee in slight flexion and the foot in the corrected position for six weeks. A below-the-knee cast is sufficient if the tendo Achilles is not lengthened or if the tibialis anterior is not transferred.

In rare cases when calluses form under the head of the second metatarsal, it is advisable to remove a dorsal wedge of bone from the base of the second metatarsal as well as from the first metatarsal. Only in one case in his experience did Dr Cooper find an indication for a lateral closing-wedge osteotomy of the calcaneus as described by Dwyer. In most cases this operation is not necessary since a few degrees of heel varus are compatible with a normal gait. The long-term results of Cooper's procedures performed over thirty years are very gratifying. They will be published by Dr Cooper (Figs 42A and 42B).

Triple arthrodesis
A triple arthrodesis is a salvage procedure to be done in children over 9 or 10 years of age with a rigid cavovarus deformity. These patients have large calluses on the lateral aspect of the sole of the foot, particularly under the base of the fifth metatarsal, and often under the head of the first metatarsal. The triple arthrodesis is indicated when the ankle joint motion is fairly good but the tarsal joints are very rigid in supination.

The operation is done through a lateral incision from the tip of the lateral malleolus to the base of the fourth metatarsal. The skin, the subcutaneus tissue, and a portion of the inferior extensor retinaculum are incised. The branches of the sural and musculocutaneus nerves are preserved and retracted with the deep fascia to expose the extensor digitorum brevis. This muscle is detached from the calcaneus and reflected forward. The tendons of the peroneus tertius and the extensor digitorum longus are retracted forwards. The inferior peroneal retinaculum with the peroneal tendons are retracted downward. After stripping the joint capsules, the calcaneocuboid and the talonavicular joints are clearly exposed (Fig. 43). The cartilage of these joints is removed with a sharp osteotome taking only a minimal amount of subchondral bone. To remove all the cartilage of the talonavicular joint it is helpful to pass a Kocher retractor along the joint margin while lifting the joint capsule. A Kocher retractor is

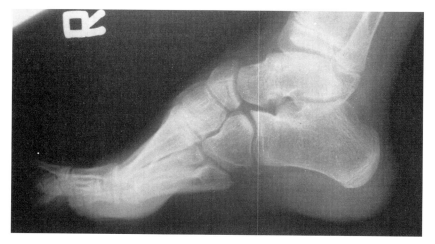

A

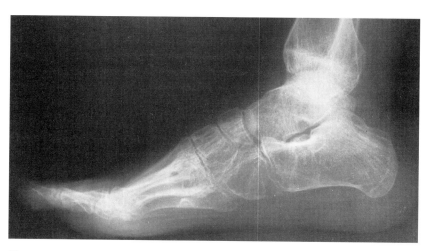

B

Fig. 42A and 42B Lateral roentgenograms of the right foot of a 13-year-old girl with congenital clubfeet and arthrogryposis involving both feet and the left hand. The feet were treated with manipulations and plaster cast changes weekly for 6 weeks starting at 4 days of age, and for 6 more weeks at 4 months of age and again at 18 months of age when the tendo Achilles was lengthened. A medial release operation was done at 3 years of age and again at 6 years of age to treat relapses. A cavovarus deformity developed in the right foot. The roentgenograms above were taken at 13 years of age before **A** and 2 months after **B** Cooper procedures to treat the cavovarus deformity (see text). The deformity did not relapse and the patient walked well when seen 6 years after the operation.

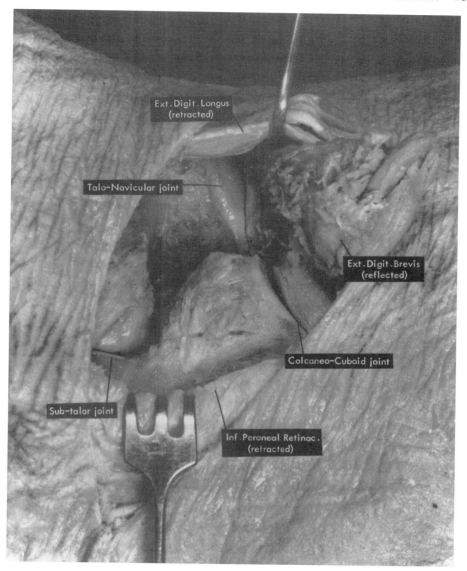

Fig. 43 Surgical exposure of the hindfoot joints (see text). (From R. Consentino 1960: *Altas of anatomy and surgical approaches in orthopaedic surgery*. Charles C. Thomas, Springfield, IL.)

now inserted around the lateral and posterior margins of the posterior talocalcaneal joints stripping the capsular insertions and fully exposing the joint. The cartilage and a minimal amount of subcondral bone is removed with a sharp osteotome. The calcaneus is separated from the talus and the interosseous talocalcaneal ligaments are thoroughly removed. The cartilage of the medial talocalcaneal joint is removed while care is taken not to injure the sustentaculum tali and the neurovascular and tendon structures of the medial aspect of the foot. A medial incision is not necessary.

Only the joint cartilage and a minimal amount of subchondral bone has to be removed from the three joints to facilitate the lateral displacement and abduction of the navicular, cuboid, and calcaneus necessary to correct the heel varus and the tarsal supination. No fixation is required and the the foot remains stable in the corrected position. After suturing the extensor digitorum brevis to the inferior peroneal retinaculum the wound is closed in layers. The foot is immobilized in the neutral position in a short-leg plaster cast. The cast is worn

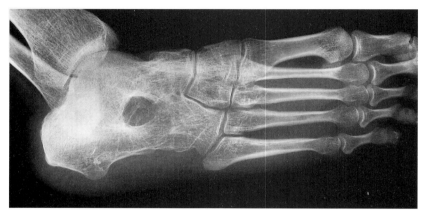

A

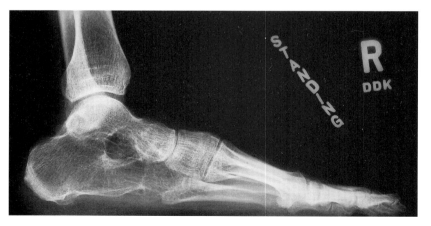

B

Figs 44A and 44B Roentgenograms of the right foot of a 37-year-old man with cerebral palsy who had a triple arthrodesis at 14 years of age to correct a clubfoot deformity.

without weight-bearing for four weeks. Another very-well-molded walking plaster cast is applied for six more weeks (Figs 44A and 44B).

Bone-wedge resections are unnecessary to correct varus deformities of the hindfoot. Indeed, a clear understanding of how the heel varus and foot supination of a clubfoot should be corrected at any age is gained when a triple arthrodesis is properly performed. The wrong technique is described and illustrated in most orthopedic textbooks: wedges of bone are removed from the lateral aspect of the midtarsal and subtalar joints, gaps are closed by abducting the foot and everting the heel, and staples are used to maintain the correction. This incorrect technique illustrates the common misunderstanding that heel varus is corrected by everting the calcaneus instead of abducting (externally rotating) it under the talus, and that hindfoot varus is corrected by everting the midfoot at the Chopart's line rather than by displacing the navicular laterally in front of the head of the talus, and the cuboid in front of the abducted calcaneus. This misunderstanding interferes, even to the present day, with the correct technique for a triple arthrodesis as well as with the successful manipulative treatment of the clubfoot.

To correct the cavus after a triple arthrodesis, a dorsal wedge of bone is resected from the base of the first metatarsal, and the extensor hallucis longus tendon is transferred to the first metatarsal, as previously described.

Tibial osteotomies to internally or externally rotate the foot should never be necessary.

Talectomy

Talectomy is indicated for the treatment of very stiff clubfeet with little or no ankle motion that have relapsed after extensive tarsal release operations. The operation gives satisfactory results when performed between one and six years of age. Talectomy can be a primary surgical procedure in patients with severe clubfeet and poor or absent leg muscles suffering from arthrogryposis or mylomeningocele. The operation is performed after improving as much as possible the alignment of the foot with weekly manipulations and casting for a period not to exceed two or three months.

Removal of the talus is a safe operation because it decompresses the hindfoot and allows for the correction of the supination and the equinus deformities without stretching the nerves or the vessels. The foot is stabilized by pushing the foot backwards so that the heel is forced into its normal, posterior, prominent position. This procedure results in a plantigrade foot that articulates with limited motion between the ankle mortice and the anterior aspect of the subtalar foot plate. The foot is functional and not painful. Relapses of the deformity are rare (Menelaus 1971).

The approach for the talectomy is the same as for the tripple arthrodesis. The head of the talus appears prominent laterally because the navicular and the calcaneus are in severe adduction. All the ligaments and joint capsules inserting into the talus are severed with tenotomy scissors to avoid damaging the joint cartilage of the adjacent joints. The talus is grasped with a large towel clipp and the foot is manipulated into equinus and supination so that the posterior and medial ligaments can be clearly seen while they are being divided. To facilitate the posterior displacement of the foot, the deltoid, spring, and posterior ankle ligaments as well as the tip of the lateral malleolus should be resected. The ankle mortice should fit into the anterior upper surface of the calcaneus. The lateral surface of the lateral malleolus below the growth plate should be trimmed to narrow the ankle and facilitate shoeing. A Steinman pin is inserted upwards through the calcaneus into the tibia to maintain the foot posteriorly in the proper position with respect to the tibia.

The foot is immobilized in a few degrees of plantar flexion in a short-leg cast. The cast and the Steinman pin are removed four weeks later and another well-molded walking plaster cast is applied for six more weeks. A well-molded leg brace is worn for 6 more months to prevent relapses of the deformity.

References

Aronson, J. and Puskarich, C.L. (1990). Deformity and disability from treated clubfoot. *J. Pediatr. Orthop.*, **10**, 109.

Attlee, J.L. (1868). *A practical manual of the treatment of clubfeet*. Appleton, New York. 1868

Browne, D. (1934). Talipes equinovarus. *Lancet*, **2**, 969.

Carroll, N.C. (1987). Congenital clubfoot. Pathoanatomy and treatment. *Instructional Course Lectures*, **36**, 117.

Coleman, S.S. (1987). *Complex foot deformities in children*. Lea & Febiger, Philadelphia.

Cummings, R.J., Hay, R.M., McCluskey, W.P., Mazur, J.M., and Lovell, W.W. (1994). Can clubfeet be evaluated accurately and reproducibly? In *The clubfoot*. (ed. G.W. Simons), Springer-Verlag, New York.

Dimeglio, A. (1977). Le traitement chirurgicale du pied bot varus equin. *Encyclopedie medico chirurgicale*. Tome Techniques Chirurgicales, Paris.

Epeldegui, T. (1993). *Conceptos y controversias sobre el pie zambo*. Vincente ed, Madrid.

Huson, A. (1961). Een outleed kundig functioneel Ouderzoek van der Voetwortel (An anatomical and functional study of the tarsus). PhD dissertation, Leiden University.

Huson, A. (1991). Functional anatomy of the foot. In *Disorders of the foot and ankle*, (2nd edn), (ed. J.H. Jahss), Vol. 1. W.B. Saunders, Philadelphia.

Hutchins, P.M., foster, B.K., Paterson, D.C., and Cole, E.A. (1985). The long term results of early surgical release in clubfeet. *J. Bone Joint Surg.*, **67B**, 791.

Hutchins, P.M., Rambick, D., Comacchio, L., and Paterson, D.C. (1986). Tibiofibular torsion in normal and treated clubfoot populations. *J. Pediatr. Orthop.*, **6**, 452.

Inman, V.T. (1976). *Inman's joints of the ankle*. Williams & Wilkins, Baltimore.

Ionasescu, V., Maynard, J.A., Ponseti, I.V., and Zellweger, H. (1974). The role of collagen in the pathogenesis of idiopathic clubfoot. Biochemical and electron microscopic correlations. *Helv. Paediat. Acta*, **29**, 305.

Kite, J.H. (1930). Non-operative treatment of congenital clubfeet. *Southern Med. J.*, **23**, 337.

Kite, J.H. (1964). *The clubfoot*. Grune & Stratton, New York London.

Kite, J.H. (1963). Some suggestions on the treatment of clubfoot by casts. AAOS Instructional Course Lecture. *J. Bone Joint Surg.*, **45A**, 406.

Krishna, M., Evans, R., Taylor, J.F., and Theis, J.C. (1991). Tibial torsion measured by ultrasound in children with talipes equinovarus. *J. Bone Joint Surg.*, **73B**, 207.

Laaveg, S.J. and Ponseti, I.V. (1980). Long-term results of treatment of congenital clubfeet. *J. Bone Joint Surg.*, **62A**, 23.

LeNoir, J.L. (1966). *Congenital idiopathic talipes*. Charles C. Thomas, Springfield, IL.

Menelaus, M.B. (1971). Talectomy for equinovarus deformity in arthrogryposis and spina bifida. *J. Bone Joint Surg.*, **53B**, 468.

Neil, H. (1825). *A practical manual of the treatment of clubfeet*. Appleton, New York.

Rose, G.K., Welton, E.A., and Marshall, T. (1985). The diagnosis of flat foot in the child. *J. Bone Joint Surg.*, **67B**, 71.

Sayre, L.A. (1875). *A practical manual of the treatment of clubfeet*. Appleton, (ed.) New York.

Stark, J.G., Johanson, J.E., and Winter, R.B. (1987). The Heyman–Herndon tarsometatarsal capsulotomy for metatarsus adductus: results in 48 feet. *J. Pediatr. Orthop.*, **7**, 305.

Swann, M., Lloyd-Roberts, G.C., and Catterall, A. (1969). The anatomy of uncorrected clubfeet. A study of rotation deformity. *J. Bone Joint Surg.*, **51B**, 263.

Steindler, A. (1920). Stripping of the os calcis. *J. Orthop. Surg.*, **2**, 8.

Steindler, A. (1951). *Postgraduate lectures on orthopaedic diagnosis and indications*. Charles C. Thomas, Springfield, IL.

8
Relapses

Regardless of the mode of treatment, the clubfoot has a stubborn tendency to relapse. It is wrongly assumed that relapses occur because the deformity has not been completely corrected. Actually, relapses are caused by the same pathology that initiated the deformity. Stiff, severe clubfeet with a small calf size are more prone to relapse than less severe feet. Unless splinted, relapses occur swiftly in premature infants, and more slowly later on. Relapses are rare after 5 years of age and extremely rare after 7 years of age regardless of whether the deformity is fully or partially corrected.

Post-correction splints with well-fitted high-top shoes attached in external rotation to a bar worn for three to four years at night, as earlier indicated, is an indispensable part of our treatment. Within similar degrees of severity a relapse is less likely in a cooperative child with responsible parents who follow instructions faithfully. About half of the recurrences are observed from 2 to 4 months after the splints are discarded, usually on the family's own initiative, when the parents see that the feet look normal when the child walks and yield to the child's resistance to continuing to wear the night splints.

In the first twenty years of our treatment, relapses occurred in about half of the patients at ages ranging from 10 months to 5 years with two and a half years as an average (Ponseti and Smoley 1983). In the last twenty years relapses have been less frequent, since there has been greater awareness on the part of parents of the importance of using night splints after correction.

A relapse is detected when there is an appearance of a slight equinus and varus deformity of the heel, often without increased adduction and cavus deformities of the forefoot. In most of our cases forefoot correction was permanent. The adduction of the forefoot relapsed to less than 20 degrees in fewer than one-fourth of our cases. It was easily corrected by manipulations and two to three plaster casts. I have observed a severe relapse of the forefoot adduction in two cases only. These were corrected by capsulotomies at the Lisfranc line, resulting in stiffness and pain in adult life as also reported by others (Stark *et al.* 1987).

The relapse of the cavus deformity is usually mild and responds well to manipulation and plaster casts with upward pressure applied on the first metatarsal head. A subcutaneous plantar fasciotomy is rarely necessary (only in 6 per cent of the cases). A recession of the extensor hallucis longus tendon to the neck of the first metatarsal may be performed, if needed, to correct severe plantar flexion of the first metatarsal.

The more important relapses occur in the hindfoot and appear to be related to the retraction of the posterior and medial ankle and tarsal ligaments and musculo-tendinous units owing to the same pathology that caused the original deformity (see chapter 5, Pathogenesis). However, surgically treated clubfeet, in which at least part of the retracted ligaments are removed and the tendons are lengthened, frequently relapse as well (Goldner and Fitch 1994), presumably owing to the retracting surgical scar tissue and persistent muscle fibrosis.

In general, the original correction may be recovered in four to six weeks with manipulations and plaster casts, changed every fourteen days, holding the foot in marked external rotation and as much dorsiflexion as possible at the ankle. This treatment is followed by lengthening the tendo Achilles when dorsiflexion of the ankle is less than 15 degrees. The last plaster cast is left on for three to four weeks. When the cast is removed, shoes attached in external rotation to a bar are worn at night until the child is about 4 years old.

To prevent further relapses, the tendon of the tibialis anterior muscle is transferred to the third cuneiform in children over $2\frac{1}{2}$ years of age if this muscle tends to strongly supinate the foot. This supination often takes place when the medial navicular displacement is not fully corrected and the AP talocalcaneal angle is under 20 degrees. Transfer of the tibialis anterior tendon averts further relapses, maintains the correction of the heel varus, improves the anteroposterior talocalcaneal angle, and thus greatly reduces the need for medial release operations. The tibialis anterior tendon transfer is an easier operation which is much less damaging to the foot than the release of the tarsal joints. Joint releases are needed when the deformity recurs in spite of the tibialis anterior transfer. The tibialis anterior tendon should never be split so as not to lose its eversion power, nor should it be transferred to the fifth metatarsal or to the cuboid since this may excessively evert the foot causing severe foot pronation and heel valgus.

The following two cases will serve as illustration:

The bilateral clubfeet of a seven-month-old premature baby girl were corrected in one month with manipulation and four plaster cast changes. When the last casts were removed no shoes were available for bracing the tiny feet (Figs 45A, 45B, and 45C). So we asked the mother to bring the baby back to the clinic in a week for custom-made shoes. To my surprise, the deformity had recurred to almost the same degree as it was originally (Figs 45D and 45E). This time the clubfeet were corrected with manipulation and three plaster casts. After correction a splint was applied which the parents discarded after one week. Three months later the deformity had recurred to a minimal degree in the right foot and only to 20 degrees of supination in the left foot. Although anatomically less severe, this time the relapsed feet were more rigid. Thus, speed of relapse slowed considerably a few weeks after birth. The feet were again corrected with manipulations and three plaster cast changes. This time the parents kept the splints on the baby for 2 months full-time and then at night only. At 14 months of age the feet appeared normal and the baby walked well (Figs 45F and 45G). She will wear the splints at night for at least another year.

The severe clubfeet of a 1-month-old baby boy were corrected in two and a half months with seven plaster casts and heel cord tenotomies (Figs 46A and 46B). A splint was worn full time for three months and, at night, for four years. At five years of age the feet remained corrected (Fig. 46C). On his next visit two years later, the deformity had relapsed in both feet (Fig. 46D). The relapse was severe in the right foot necessitating three corrective toe-to-groin plaster casts and a transfer of the tibialis anterior to the third cuneiform. The relapse was less severe in the left foot. It was corrected after applying three plaster casts (Fig. 46E). At 35 years of age his feet were plantigrade, painless, and functioned well.

In the left foot the heel was in 5 degrees of varus and the plantar arch was higher than the right (Figs 46F, 46G, 46H, and 46I). The talocalcaneal angle measured 16 degrees on the right and 14 degrees on the left. The navicular was slightly medially displaced worse on the right.

References

Goldner, J.L. and Fitch, R.D. (1994). Classification and evaluation of congenital talipes equinovarus. In, *The clubfoot*, (ed. G.W. Simons). Springer-Verlag, New York.

Ponseti, I.V. and Smoley, E.N. (1983). Congenital club foot: the results of treatment. *J. Bone Joint Surg.*, **45A**, 261.

Stark, J.G., Johanson, J.E., and Winter, R.B. (1987). The Heyman–Herndon tarsometatarsal capsulotomy for metatarsus adductus: results in 48 patients. *J. Pediatr. Orthop.*, **7**, 305.

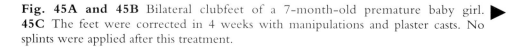

Fig. 45A and 45B Bilateral clubfeet of a 7-month-old premature baby girl. ▶ **45C** The feet were corrected in 4 weeks with manipulations and plaster casts. No splints were applied after this treatment.

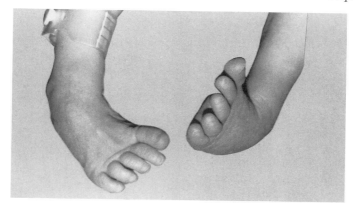

A

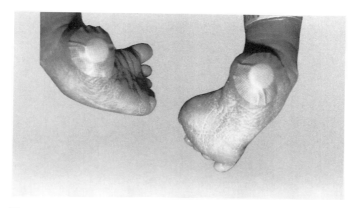

B

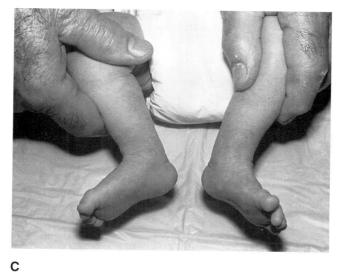

C

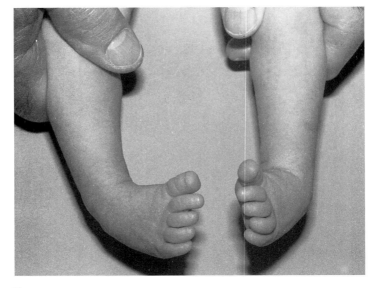

D

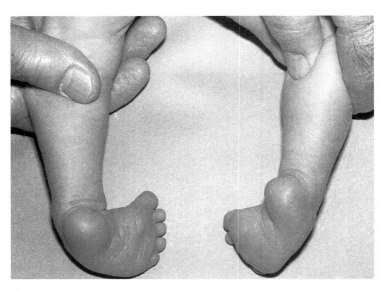

E

Fig. 45D and 45E The deformity relapsed in one week.

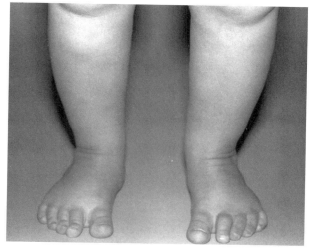

F

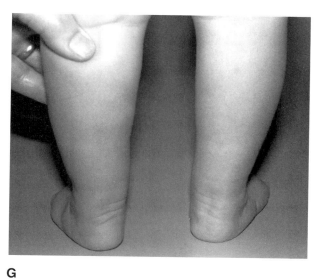

G

Fig. 45F and 45G At 14 months of age the feet look normal and the child walks well (see text).

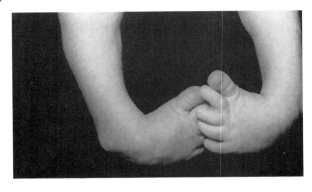

A

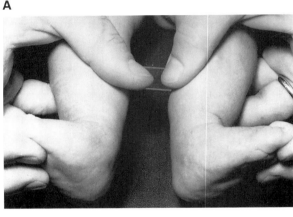

B

Fig. 46A and 46B The clubfeet of a 1-month-old baby (A) were corrected in two and a half months (B).

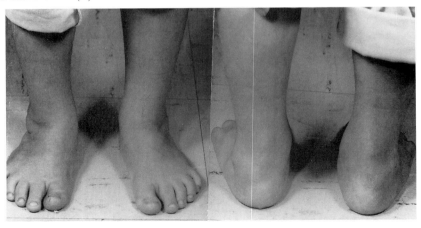

C

Fig. 46C At 5 years of age the feet remain corrected.

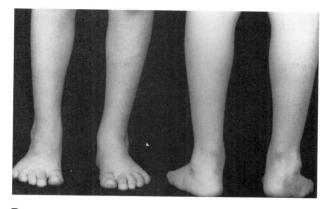

D

Fig. 46D At 7 years of age the deformity had relapsed in both feet and was treated as explained in the text.

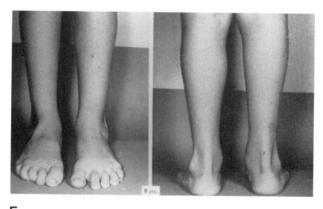

E

Fig. 46E At 8 years of age the feet were well corrected.

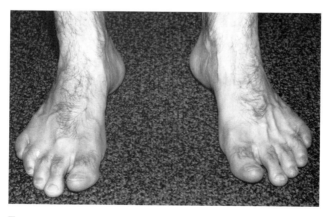

F

Fig. 46F At 35 years of age the feet are plantigrade, painless, and function well.

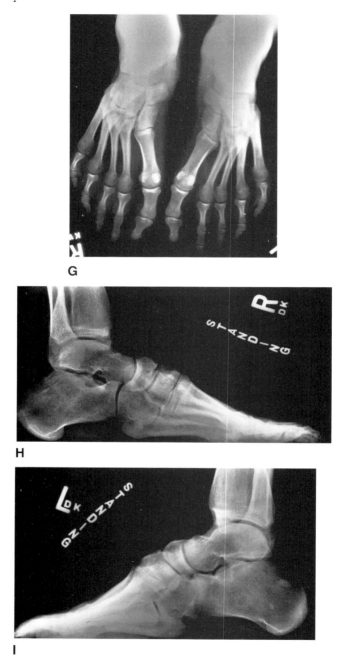

G

H

I

Fig. 46G, 46H, and 46I Anteroposterior and lateral roentgenograms of both feet show some cavus on the left and smaller than normal talocalcaneal angles. In the anteroposterior roentgenograms the profiles of the first cuneiform–first metatarsal joints are in a posteromedially inclined plane. The joint spaces are of normal width.

9
Outcomes of treatment

Evaluation of functional results of clubfoot treatment necessitates follow-ups into adult life. Results of follow-up studies before adolescence are not very meaningful because most children with defective feet do not complain; their endurance and activity are boundless. Joint stiffness and muscle weakness are not as limiting in children as they are in adults. Clinical results cannot be evaluated before at least five years of age when relapses become infrequent.

A large sample of the severe cases of clubfeet treated by us from infancy have been studied for evaluation on four occasions. Included in our follow-up studies are patients with feet necessitating four or more plaster cast changes for their correction. Mild cases of foot deformity have not been included in any of our follow-up studies. Some patients are included in each of the four studies, while others, those who did not return to Iowa City for evaluation, are not.

The first evaluation, by Eugene N. Smoley and myself, of patients treated from 1948 to 1956 was published in 1963. From 1948 to 1956 we treated 286 cases of clubfoot in otherwise normal children. Not included in our study were 149 patients originally treated in other clinics and referred to us for further correction, and 46 patients with mild clubfeet corrected by simple manipulations and the application of one to three plaster clasts. Of the remaining 91 patients with severe untreated clubfeet 24 were lost to follow-up. We were, therefore, able to evaluate the results of treatment in 67 patients with a total of 94 clubfeet. The age of the patients at the onset of treatment ranged from one week to six months, the average being one month. Many variations in the degree of rigidity were present. From five to ten (average 7.6) plaster casts worn for periods of 5 to 12 weeks (average 9.5 weeks) were necessary for the correction of all the clubfoot components. In 74 of the 94 feet the tendo Achilles was sectioned subcutaneously. Anteroposterior and lateral roentgenograms and photographs of the feet of all patients were made before treatment, after the removal of the last plaster cast, and at the last clinical evaluation; the latter took place five to thirteen years after the initial treatment.

In 53 feet (56 per cent) the deformity recurred one or more times and required further treatment. A relapse of the equinus was observed in 18 feet. In eight of these feet, the tendo Achilles had been sectioned during the initial treatment. The relapses were treated with a second percutaneous section of the tendo Achilles in ten feet and with a formal tendo Achilles lengthening in eight feet. A transfer of the tibialis anterior tendon to the dorsum of the foot was performed in 39 of the feet after the second or third recurrence. The operation was successful in 30 feet, but from 1 to 10 degrees of heel varus persisted in nine feet. The nine failures of the anterior tibial tendon transfer to correct the varus deformity of the heel could be blamed on surgical errors (broken wires, loosening of the silk stitches, wrong site of insertion). Excessive plantar flexion of the first metatarsal or cock-up of the big toe was observed in six feet. These deformities occurred before the transfer in three feet and after the transfer in three other feet. A medial release operation was done in one foot after the second recurrence and in two feet after the third recurrence.

The cavus deformity recurred in six feet. A subcutaneous plantar fasciotomy was done in three feet. The extensor hallucis longus was transferred to the neck of the first metatarsal in three other feet. One foot had a severe recurrence of the forefoot adduction and was treated by capsulotomies at the Lisfranc line. This operation caused severe foot stiffness.

Out of the 94 feet studied, the clubfoot deformity was well corrected clinically and roentgenographically in 67 feet (71 per cent); 26 feet had a residual heel varus of 0 to 10 degrees and only 0 to 10 degrees of ankle dorsiflexion. One foot had a poor result with 12 degrees of heel varus and 22 degrees of forefoot adduction. None of the children had pain and all could walk on their toes.

In a second study, by Dr Jerónimo Campos and myself, (Ponseti and Campos 1972), we reported further observations on our clubfoot treatment, mostly addressing the effect of the tibialis anterior tendon transfer on the permanence of the correction. We examined and took roentgenograms of the feet of 34 patients between 9 and 20 years of age (average 16 years), with a total of 58 operated feet. Of these, 43 feet had a transfer of the tibialis anterior tendon to the third cuneiform and 15 to the cuboid. This transfer to the cuboid caused overcorrection in 10 feet, and in two of these with severe planovalgus the tendon had to be retransferred to the second cuneiform in addition to having a Grice bone block (Grice 1952). Of the 43 feet with the tendon transfer to the third cuneiform, four had a persistent supination that was treated with medial soft-tissue release one to three years following the transfer. One of these feet had a triple arthrodesis 10 years later. Thirty-three feet were well aligned. In 15 feet the heel was in less than 10 degrees of varus. In ten feet the heel was in less than 10 degrees of valgus. The forefoot was well corrected in all but three feet which had 10 to 20 degrees of adduction. A tendency to cock-up deformity of the big toe was observed in 12 feet. None of the patients had pain or complaints about their feet. Most of them were participating in high school athletics. All could walk on their toes. Some joint stiffness and muscle weakness were observed in the feet treated with medial soft-tissue releases.

A third study, by Sterling J. Laaveg, of 70 patients with 104 clubfeet treated under my direction and followed for 10 to 27 years after treatment, was published in 1980. We chose patients who were less than 6 months old when first seen and who had no previous treatment elsewhere. The mean age at follow-up was 18.8 years. The aim was to determine whether our treatment gave the patient a functional, painless foot. We attempted to correlate the patients' opinion of the appearance and function of the treated clubfeet with both the method of treatment and roentgenographic findings.

Of the 104 clubfeet, 13 were treated with manipulation and plaster casts only; 42 were treated with plaster casts and lengthening of the tendo Achilles (93 per cent of the lengthenings were done subcutaneously under local anesthesia); 48 were treated with a transfer of the tibialis anterior tendon to the third cuneiform bone; and one was treated with a transfer of the tibialis posterior tendon to the dorsum of the foot through the interosseous membrane. Of the 48 feet treated by transfer of the tibialis anterior tendon, two had no other procedure; 29 also had lengthening of the tendo Achilles; and 17 had a variety of surgical procedures including recession of the extensor hallucis longus tendon to the neck of the first metatarsal (ten feet), plantar fasciotomy (six feet), posteromedial release (four feet), posterior release of the ankle and subtalar joints (three feet), transfer of the extensor digitorum communis tendon to the metatarsals (three feet), and triple arthrodesis (two feet).

The mean age of the 70 patients at the beginning of treatment was 6.9 weeks; the mean number of casts used during their initial treatment was seven; the mean duration of the initial treatment with plaster casts was 8.6 weeks; the mean number of casts used for all treatment (initial treatment and treatment of relapses) was nine; and the mean time of night-splint use was 49.5 months.

Fifty-five (53 per cent) of the clubfeet had no relapse; 49 (47 per cent) had one relapse at a mean age of 39 months; 25 had a second relapse at a mean age of 53 months; ten had a third relapse at a mean age of 63 months; and three had a fourth relapse at a mean age of 77 months.

Each patient in the study filled out a questionnaire requesting information relative to his/her level of activity, participation in sports, foot pain, problems with shoes, appearance of the foot, and satisfaction with the final result. All 70 patients had an orthopedic and neurological examination in which the strength of the muscles of the thigh, leg, and foot were recorded, along with stance, gait, and motion of the ankle and foot. The limb length, circumference of the leg, and length and width of the foot were measured. A force-plate analysis was done to determine the location of the resultant foot–floor reaction force for both feet during gait.

Anteroposterior and lateral roentgenograms of the feet were made with the patient standing. On the AP roentgenograms, we measured the anteroposterior talocalcaneal angle and the angle between the longitudinal axes of the calcaneus and fifth metatarsal, according to the method of Beatson and Pearson (1966). Using the same method on the lateral roentgenograms, we measured the lateral talocalcaneal angle and the angle between the longitudinal axes of the first and fifth metatarsals. We calculated the talocalcaneal index, which is the sum of the anteroposterior and lateral talocalcaneal angles as described by Beatson and Pearson. The anteroposterior talocalcaneal angle reflects the varus–valgus position of the heel; the anteroposterior angle between the calcaneus and the fifth metatarsal measures the degree of metatarsus adductus; the lateral angle between the first and fifth metatarsals shows the degree of pes cavus.

The normal feet of the 28 patients with unilateral deformity were used as controls. We compared the clinical and roentgenographic variables in all of the normal feet and in all of the clubfeet. The rating of function and the patients' satisfaction with the results as indicated by their response to the questionnaire were each correlated with the patient's age at initial treatment, the total number of plaster casts, the number of relapses, the degree of ankle dorsiflexion, the degree of foot pronation and supination, the position of the heel, the adduction of the anterior part of the foot while standing, the anteroposterior and lateral talocalcaneal angles, and the talocalcaneal index. Significant correlations were identified by the *t*-test at 0.05 level of significance.

In all of the patients with unilateral clubfoot, the normal foot was longer and wider than the clubfoot and the circumference of the leg was greater on the normal side than on the side with the clubfoot. The limb lengths, on the other hand, were the same. The mean difference between the lengths of the feet was 1.3 cm; between the widths of the feet, 0.4 cm; and between the circumferences of the legs, 2.3 cm.

A rating system for functional results was designed, with 100 points indicating a normal foot. These included a maximum score of 30 points for amount of pain; 20 points each for level of activity and patient satisfaction; and 10 points each for motion of the ankle and foot, and position of the heel during stance and gait (Table 2).

The results were classified according to the scores, as follows: excellent, 90 to 100 points; good, 80 to 89 points; fair 70 to 79; and poor, less than 70 points. The results were rated excellent in 54 per cent of the feet, good in 20 per cent, fair in 14 per cent, and poor in 12 per cent.

The mean rating of function for all 104 clubfeet was 87.5 points, with a standard deviation of 11.7 points and a range of 50 to 100 points. The mean ratings for the feet treated with plaster casts only was 93.9 points; for those treated with plaster casts and tendo Achilles lengthening it was 92.4 points; for the feet treated by plaster casts, tendo Achilles lengthening, and transfer of the tibialis anterior tendon it was 80.5 points, a much lower rating than the mean ratings of all the other feet. As might be expected, the results were not as good in the more resistent clubfeet requiring further treatment.

Fifty-nine per cent of the 70 patients stated that their corrected clubfeet were never painful, 24 per cent had occasional mild pain after strenuous activities, and 9 per cent had occasional pain during routine activities. None of the 104 patients experienced pain when walking. Seventy-two per cent had no limitation of activity, and 18 per cent had mild limitation of activity. Eighty-nine per cent stated that their corrected clubfoot was normal or close to normal in appearance, and 99 per cent were able to wear normal shoes of the same size.

Table 2 Functional rating system for clubfoot

Category	Points
Satisfaction (20 points)	
I am	
(a) very satisfied with the end result	20
(b) satisfied with the end result	16
(c) neither satisfied nor unsatisfied with the end result	12
(d) unsatisfied with the end result	8
(e) very unsatisfied with the end result	4
Function (20 points)	
In my daily living, my club foot	
(a) does not limit my activities	20
(b) occasionally limits my strenuous activities	16
(c) usually limits me in strenuous activities	12
(d) limits me occasionally in routine activities	8
(e) limits me in walking	4
Pain (30 points)	
My club foot	
(a) is never painful	30
(b) occasionally causes mild pain during strenuous activities	24
(c) usually is painful after strenuous activities only	18
(d) is occasionally painful during routine activities	12
(e) is painful during walking	6
Position of heel when standing (10 points)	
Heel varus, 0° or some heel valgus	10
Heel varus, 1–5°	5
Heel varus, 6–10°	3
Heel varus, greater than 10°	0
Passive motion (10 points)	
Dorsiflexion	1 point per 5° (up to 5 points)
Total varus–valgus motion of heel	1 point per 10° (up to 3 points)
Total anterior inversion–eversion of foot	1 point per 25° (up to 2 points)
Gait (10 points)	
Normal	6
Can toe-walk	2
Can heel-walk	2
Limp	−2
No heel-strike	−2
Abnormal toe-off	−2

Seventy-two per cent of the patients were very satisfied with the end result of their treatment, 19 per cent were satisfied, and only 4 per cent were not satisfied.

The mean amounts of dorsiflexion of the ankle (31 degrees in the normal feet; 13 degrees in the clubfeet), varus–valgus motion of the heel (39 degrees in the normal feet; 26.8 degrees in the clubfeet), and inversion–eversion of the anterior part of the foot (65 degrees in the normal feet; 52.1 degrees in the clubfeet) were between one and two standard deviations lower in the limbs with the corrected clubfeet than in the normal limbs. The feet that were treated by tibialis anterior tendon transfer had significantly less motion than those without the transfer. The mean position of the heel in the clubfeet while standing was one degree of valgus deviation, and no significant difference was found between the two groups. The mean metatarsus adductus while standing was 2.8 degrees.

All 70 patients could walk without limping and could also walk on their toes. The cavus was completely corrected in 90 per cent of the feet while 10 per cent retained a mild cavus. A low functional rating correlated with decreased dorsiflexion of the ankle, and with the inversion–eversion motion of the forepart of the foot.

The roentgenograms of the treated clubfeet revealed that the mean values for the anteroposterior talocalcaneal angle (14.5 degrees), lateral talocalcaneal angle (20.9 degrees), and talocalcaneal index (36.5 degrees) were at least one standard deviation less than the corresponding mean values in the normal feet (20, 25, and 53 degrees, respectively). There were no significant differences among the mean anteroposterior talocalcaneal angles and talocalcaneal indexes of the feet with excellent, good, fair, and poor functional ratings. The mean lateral talocalcaneal angles, on the other hand were significantly different in each group rating. In the normal feet the mean lateral angle was 33 degrees; in the corrected feet rated excellent, the mean lateral angle was 22.4 degrees; in those rated good it was 20.5 degrees; in fair, 18.4 degrees; and in poor, 17.4 degrees. The functional rating and the patient's satisfaction correlated highly with the ranges of motion of the ankle and foot, the appearance of the foot, the amount of pain, the level of activity, and the lateral talocalcaneal angle.

A force-plate analysis of our subjects was done in the Orthopedic Biomechanics Laboratories under the direction of Dr Richard A. Brand to compare the center-of-pressure path, that is, the location of the vertical foot-floor contact force resultant during gait in normal subjects and in those with corrected clubfeet (Brand *et al.* 1981). From the group of patients studied by Laaveg and myself, 44 subjects ranging from 13 to 26 years of age (average 20.6 years) were randomly selected. Center-of-pressure paths during gait were determined with a Kistler piezoelectric force-plate. This device, together with a PDP-12 computer, determined the location of the resultant vertical foot–floor contact force. Harris footmats were placed on the force-plate and subjects were instructed to walk barefoot across the plate at a comfortable pace.

The center-of-pressure paths were superimposed for normal subjects and for patients with corrected clubfeet having various functional ratings. We also plotted the center of pressure paths for those subjects who had the smallest lateral talocalcaneal angles (average 16 degrees) and the smallest anteroposterior talocalcaneal angles (average 7 degrees).

Our studies in normal adults demonstrate fairly constant foot–floor contact area shapes and confirm the previous observation that the center-of-pressure path is fairly constant in normal feet. All treated clubfeet were plantigrade, and, even though the foot–floor contact areas were wider than those of the normal feet, the center-of-pressure paths were generally no closer to the lateral aspect of the foot than in normal subjects. The patients did not tend to walk with the clubfeet inverted nor did they have callosities on the lateral aspect of the sole. The lower the functional results the more variable are the center-of-pressure paths within the various groups. However, some of the paths in all the functional groups appeared virtually normal, suggesting that the center-of-pressure paths do not always distinguish between normal and our treated feet. Clubfeet patients generally did not begin heel strike as far posterior as normal subjects did. This is probably owing to the limited dorsiflexion in the abnormal group.

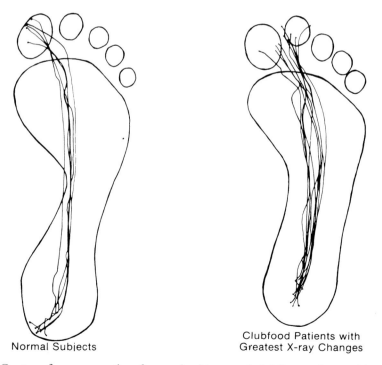

Normal Subjects   Clubfoot Patients with
                                   Greatest X-ray Changes

Fig. 47 Center of pressure paths of normal subjects and clubfoot patients with greatest X-ray changes.

There seemed to be no correlation between the radiographic result as determined by the anteroposterior or lateral talocalcaneal angles and the center-of-pressure pathways (Fig. 47). Center-of-pressure paths were not sensitive enough to be of value in distinguishing among treated patients or sometimes even between patients and normal subjects, all of whom had plantigrade feet. We did not, however, have the opportunity to study adults with severe residual deformities. It is possible that center-of-pressure paths would be grossly abnormal in such patients. The inability to distinguish clearly between patients with varying functional ratings did correlate with the fact that all our patients functioned well.

In the fourth study, conducted by Drs Douglas M. Cooper and Frederick R. Dietz in 1992–93, (see Cooper and Dietz 1995), the clubfoot patients treated in our hospital between 1950 and 1967 were contacted. Forty-five patients, 26 with bilateral clubfeet and 19 with unilateral (total 71 clubfeet) and ranging in age from 25 to 42 years (average 34 years), were able to return to our clinic for a thorough evaluation. Thirty of the 71 clubfeet had had a tibialis anterior transfer. Seventeen of these patients had been evaluated in the late seventies by Dr Laaveg and myself.

The patients were asked to fill out a questionnaire requesting information on occupation, education, pain, function, and satisfaction with the results. They underwent a thorough clinical and radiographic examination. No important change was perceived in the responses of the 17 patients to the questionnaires given in 1978 and in 1992. However, ten patients had calluses, most of them under the fourth or fifth metatarsal heads. Twelve patients had tenderness to palpation: five around the ankle joint, three along the plantar fascia, three under the metatarsal heads, and one at the tendo Achilles insertion. All patients could walk on their toes. Three could not walk on their heels due to limited dorsiflexion. The strength of all leg and foot muscles in the 71 clubfeet was rated 5 on a 5-point scale. The strength of the tibialis anterior muscle in 25 of 30 transferred tendons was also rated 5; in the other five transferred tendons it was rated 4+.

The comparison of the roentgenograms taken in the late seventies with roentgenograms of the same patients taken in 1993 indicate that only two patients had increased osteoarthritic changes. These changes consisted of slightly larger osteophytes on the dorsum of the talar neck.

Some additional tests were done during the 1993 study. An electrogoniometer (Ankle-Foot Elgon, Therapeutics Unlimited, Iowa City, Iowa) with the leads placed on the anterior proximal tibia and the navicular and second cuneiform was used to accurately measure passive and active foot and ankle motion (Fig. 48). Electrogoniometric analysis revealed a decreased passive and active dorsiflexion, plantarflexion, and inversion in the clubfeet as compared to the normal feet. Passive and active eversion were not significantly different (see Fig. 22, Chapter 4) The degree of dorsiflexion, inversion, and eversion when walking was less than in the normal feet. No difference in plantarflexion was registered between the corrected clubfeet and the normal feet. The clubfeet

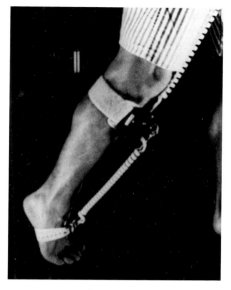

Fig. 48 Electrogoniometer to measure foot and ankle motion.

showed a mean of 9 degrees of dorsiflexion when walking, only 4 degrees less than in normal feet. Clubfeet exhibited 3 degrees less eversion and 1 degree more plantarflexion than the normal feet during gait.

To determine the overall suppleness of the foot, a digitizer was used to measure the area (square centimeters) inside the passive and active range of motion circle. The area within the passive range of motion circle was strikingly smaller in the clubfeet (29 cm^2) than in the normal feet (61 cm^2) (Fig. 49).

The patients were asked to walk on a pedobarograph (EMED-SF, Novel GMBH, Munich, Germany), a system which operates with individually calibrated capacitive pressure sensors. Values were obtained for the total area of maximum pressure (square centimeter), peak pressure of the maximum pressure picture (Newtons per square centimeter), total force normalized to body weight of the maximum pressure picture, pressure time integral (Newtons-seconds per square centimeter), and force time integral normalized to body weight. These parameters were chosen to assess different kinds of energy the foot is required to absorb. Five areas of the foot were considered: heel, midfoot, metatarsal heads, great toe, and lateral toes. Separate values were obtained for each area as well as for the entire foot. The normal feet of the 19 patients with unilateral clubfoot were the controls.

Differences between the normal feet and the clubfeet were found in specific foot regions. The heel in the clubfoot had a lesser peak pressure and total force in the maximum pressure picture when compared with normal feet. The metatarsal heads had a smaller area of maximum pressure than in normal feet.

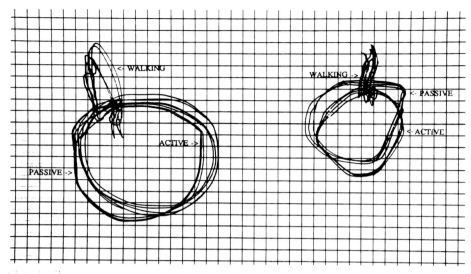

Fig. 49 The ranges of active and passive motion of a normal foot (*left*) and a treated clubfoot (*right*) as measured with the electrogoniometer show a smaller range for the clubfoot than for the normal foot. When walking, however, only a small portion of the available range of motion is needed and consequently there is no appreciable difference between the normal and the well-treated clubfoot.

Compared with normal feet, the lateral toes in clubfeet showed a larger total area of maximum pressure and a greater force time integral, suggesting a mild lateral transfer of weight bearing. These findings indicate that the limitation of dorsiflexion in clubfeet when walking results in a transfer of weight from the heel to the midfoot. That this transfer of weight is not due to a rocker-bottom deformity is supported by the fact that the arch is slightly higher as seen in the radiographs of clubfeet. None of the above-mentioned differences affects good foot function.

Since foot pain is common in adult life, Drs Cooper and Dietz wished to compare our treated patients with a group of individuals without congenital clubfoot. Ninety-seven patients in the Ophthalmology Department waiting area, who did not have congenital foot deformity and who were within the same age range as our patients, were asked to fill out a foot pain and function questionnaire identical to that completed by our study group. Based on the responses of the normal group, criteria for excellent, good, and poor function were established. An excellent foot was one that did not limit activities of daily living and was never painful or only caused mild pain occasionally. A good foot was one that occasionally limited activities of daily living or was painful after strenuous activities. A poor foot was one that limited the patient's daily activities or routine walking, or was painful during daily activities, walking, or at night.

When comparing this population with normal feet to our treated clubfoot patients the results were as follows. Sixty-two per cent of the clubfeet were excellent; 16 per cent were good; and 22 per cent were poor. In the normal subjects 63 per cent were excellent; 22 per cent were good; and 15 per cent were poor. There were no significant differences in the functional performance of our patients compared to that of a population born with normal feet. Fifty-four per cent of the clubfoot patients participated in sporting activities at least once a week compared to 40 per cent of the normal subjects. Twenty-six per cent of the clubfoot patients felt they could walk any distance without foot discomfort compared to 45 per cent of the normal patients.

The clubfoot patients were asked to stand on one foot and perform rapid toe-ups to a maximum count of forty or until they felt moderate pain or fatigue in the gastrosoleus. Fifty-two (74 per cent) of the 71 congenital clubfeet were able to do 40 rapid toe-ups compared to 94 per cent of the normal feet.

Although marked differences were present between clubfeet and normal feet on almost all measurements, very few of these differences helped discriminate between good and poor functional outcomes. Factors that showed statistically significant correlations between a good or excellent versus a poor outcome were: occupation, passive dorsiflexion measured clinically, total foot pressure time integral, and rapid toe-ups.

Occupation analysis revealed a combined 92 per cent excellent and good results versus 8 per cent poor results in the professional group compared to 60 per cent excellent and good results and 40 per cent poor results in the laborer group. It is understandable that patients whose occupations make heavy demands on their feet will experience discomfort whereas those with sedentary occupations will not.

Passive dorsiflexion measured clinically revealed 7 degrees for the excellent and good group and 4 degrees for the poor group. Pedobarograph measurements revealed that the excellent and good group had an average total foot pressure time integral of 27 Ns/cm^2 compared to 21 in the poor group. Analysis of the rapid toe-up test revealed the excellent and good group reaches an average of 38 toe-ups compared to 28 for the poor group.

All other measurements, including range of motion, pedobarographic measurements, and angles measured in the roentgenograms, did not correlate with the excellent, good, and poor outcomes. The range of motion used in walking is a fraction of the range of motion available in the normal foot. In our treated clubfeet we obtain more than the necessary range of motion needed for walking and normal activities. This explains the lack of correlation between range of motion and outcome in our treated patients whose feet, although with restricted range of motion, are fully functional.

Similarly, the lack of correlation between the outcome of our treatment and the radiographic measurements indicate that although many of our treated clubfeet are not fully corrected, the foot alignment we obtain with our treatment gives good results. Although it is important to correct the talocalcaneal

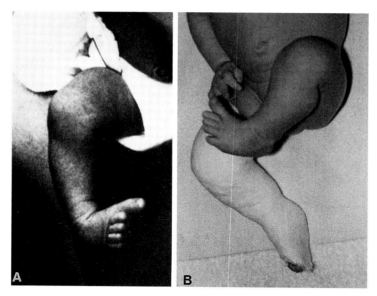

Fig. 50A Right clubfoot in a 3-week-old baby girl treated with manipulations and 6 plaster casts and a subcutaneous tenotomy of the tendo Achilles.

Fig. 50B At 4 weeks of age the right clubfoot is immobilized in a corrective plaster cast. The metatarsus adductus present at birth in the left foot has increased. It was treated with manipulations and 3 plaster casts. The child wore an external rotation splint at night for 4 years.

angles as much as possible, it is by no means necessary in order to obtain a plantigrade, well-aligned foot with good function. Certainly, a painless, well-aligned foot with good function is far better than a foot with perfectly aligned bones on the roentgenograms but with reduced range of motion owing to scarring, muscle weakness, and pain (Figs 50 and 51; and see also Fig. 46, Chapter 7).

A comparison between the results of our long-term follow-up studies of our severe cases (with the exclusion of mild cases necessitating fewer than four plaster-cast changes for correction, as earlier stated) and those of short-term follow-up studies in other clinics is not appropriate because our results address correction of the deformity emphasizing patient satisfaction and painless functional performance into adult life; our treatment is primarily manipulative with limited surgery to maintain the correction in the more severe cases. In other clinics treatment is primarily surgical including extensive joint release operations usually after a period of inadequate manipulation and cast treatment that fails to correct the deformity (Bensahel *et al.* 1987; Otremski *et al.* 1987). Furthermore, evaluation schemes 'lack a universally accepted rating system for

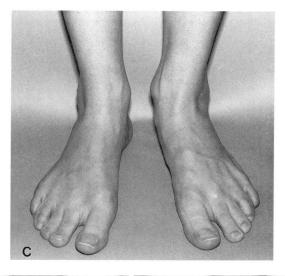

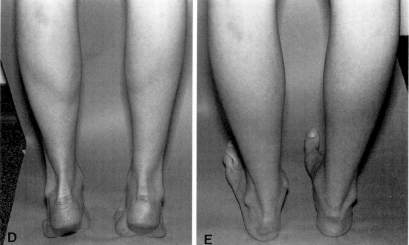

Figs 50C, 50D, and 50E At 30 years of age both feet are normal except for a slight left heel valgus. The circumference of the right calf is 1 cm smaller than the left. When standing on tip toes the smaller bulk of the right gastrocnemius raises a little higher than the left.

assessment of results' as Cummings *et al.* (1994) have warned. In addition, most follow-ups are short term and their assessment of results derives primarily from radiographic measurements and presence or absence of pain as a measure of success rather than to foot function. There is no correlation between the values of angles measured in roentgenograms and the functional results within the

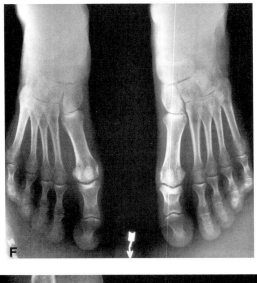

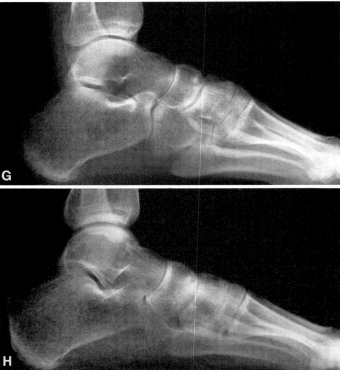

Figs 50F, 50G and 50H Standing roentgenograms of both feet. The alignment of the bones is normal. The subtalar joint in the right foot (G) is abnormal.

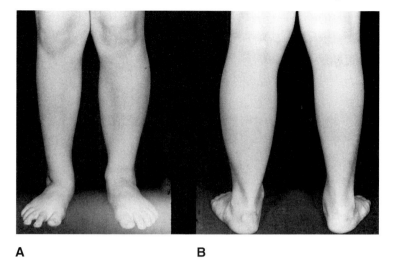

A   B

Figs 51A and 51B A 35-year-old obese woman treated at 2 weeks of age with 6 plaster casts for right congenital clubfoot. The leg with the clubfoot has much less fat than the normal leg. The circumference of the right calf is 4 cm smaller than the left. The motions of the right foot are nearly normal except for limitation of ankle dorsiflexion to the neutral position. She has no pain.

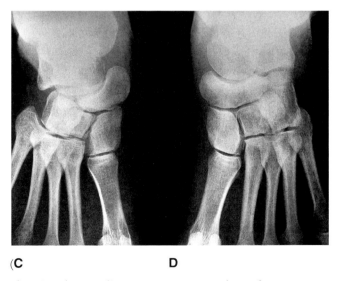

(C   D

Figs 51C and 51D The standing roentgenograms show the most severe medial displacement of the navicular in our series. The talocalcaneal angle measures 21 degrees on the right and 28 degrees on the left. On the right there is inversion of the midfoot as evidenced by the superimposition of the cuneiform and cuboid. The forefoot is in the normal position and well aligned with the hindfoot.

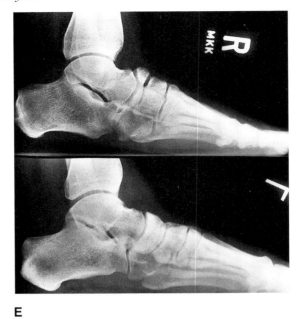

E

Fig. 51E In the lateral roentgenograms the distance between the tibia and the calcaneus in the right foot is short and the subtalar joint is very abnormal.

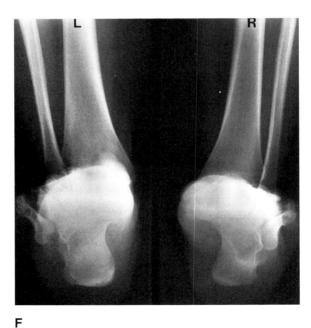

F

Fig. 51F In the hindfoot alignment view the calcaneus is in the neutral position in both feet.

range found in our treatment. Furthermore, the presence or absence of pain is not an appropriate criterium when applied to children, since pain does not usually develop even in untreated clubfeet until adolescence or later in life; and the available follow-ups do not go beyond adolescence (Turco 1981, 1994; Ricciardi-Pollini *et al.* 1984; Simons 1985; Bensahel 1990). It is regrettable that there are no long-term follow-ups of results of clubfoot surgery, although postero-medial release operations have been performed since Codivilla's time at the beginning of this century to the present day (Codivilla 1906).

In 1985, Hutchins *et al.* (1985) reported results on 252 feet treated by early posterior release followed for an average of 15 years and 10 months, the longest of the short-term follow-ups. He used our grading system and found satisfactory results in 81 per cent, of the cases but excellent and good results in only 57 per cent of the cases. He attributes the poor results to restricted ankle movement owing to the flattening of the talus. This suggests that greater bone damage may result from extensive joint releases than from careful manipulations. In 1990, Aronson *et al.* (1990) compared different types of treatment. They found that feet treated with plaster casting or casting plus tendo Achilles lengthening resulted in less deformity and disability. They also found that posteromedial release improved the talocalcaneal index but reduced both the range of motion of the ankle and the strength of plantarflexion as compared to the casting groups. These observations coincide with my experience with extensive clubfoot surgery since the forties. Our functional results and patient satisfaction improved greatly when we learned to correct clubfeet with our improved techniques of manipulation and plaster-cast treatments. Joint release operations were performed only in the very few unyielding severe cases.

No deterioration was observed in the condition of the feet in the last study when compared to the condition of the same feet studied 16 years earlier. More follow-up studies will be necessary to determine whether the condition of our treated feet worsens with aging.

References

Aronson, J. and Puskarich, Ch.L. (1990). Deformity and disability from treated club-foot. *J. Pediatr. Orthop.*, **10**, 109.

Beason, T.R. and Pearson, J.R. (1966). A method of assessing correction in club feet. *J. Bone Joint Surg.*, **48B**, 40.

Bensahel, H., Catterall, A., and Dimeglio, A. (1990). Practical applications in idiopathic clubfoot: a retrospective multicentric study in EPOS. *J. Pediatr. Orthop.*, **10**, 186.

Bensahel, H., Csukonyi, C., Desgrippes, Y., and Chaumien, J.P. (1987). Surgery in residual clubfoot. *J. Pediatr. Orthop.*, **7**, 145.

Brand, R.A., Laaveg, S.J., Crowninshield, R.D., and Ponseti, I.V. (1981). The center of pressure path in treated clubfeet. *Clin. Orthop.*, **160**, 43.

Codivilla, A. (1906). Sulla cura del piede equino-varo congenito. Nuovo metodo di cura cruenta. *Arch. Chir. Orthop.*, **23**, 254.

Cooper, D.M. and Dietz, F.R. (1995). Treatment of idiopathic clubfoot. A thirty year follow-up note. *J. Bone Joint Surg.,* **77A**, 1477.

Cummings, R.J., Hay, R.M., McCluskey, W.P., Mazur, J.M., and Lovell, W.W. (1994). Can clubfeet be evaluated accurately and reproducibily? In *The Clubfoot*, (ed. G.W. Simons), Springer-Verlag, New York.

Grice, D.S. (1952). An extra-articular arthrodesis of the subastragalar joint for correction of paralytic flat feet in children. *J. Bone Joint Surg.*, **34A**, 927.

Hutchins, P.M., Foster, B.K., Patterson, D.C., and Cole, E.A. (1980). Long term results of early surgical release in clubfeet. *J. Bone Joint Surg.*, **67B**, 791.

Laaveg, S.J. and Ponseti, I.V. (1980). Long-term results of treatment of congenital club foot. *J. Bone Joint Surg.*, **62A**, 23.

Otremski, I., Salama, R., Kermosh, O., and Weintraub, S. (1987). An analysis of the results of modified one stage posterormedial release for the treatment of clubfeet. *J. Pediatr. Orthop.*, **7**, 149.

Ponseti, IV. and Campos, J. (1972). Observations on pathogenesis and treatment of congenital clubfoot. *Clin. Orthop.*, **84**, 50.

Ponseti, I.V. and Smoley, E.N. (1963). Congenital club foot. The results of treatment. *J. Bone Joint Surg.*, **45A**, 261.

Ricciardi-Pollini, P.T., Ippolito, E., Tudisco, C., and Farsetti, P. (1984). Congenital clubfoot results of treatment of 54 cases. *Foot Ankle*, **5**, 107.

Simons, G.W. (1985) Complete subtalar release in clubfeet. Part II. *J. Bone Joint Surg.*, **67A**, 1056.

Turco, V.J. (1981). *Clubfoot*. Churchill-Livingstone, New York.

Turco, V.J (1994). Present management of idiopathic clubfoot. *J. Pediatr. Orthop.* Part B. **3**, 149.

10
Radiographic study of treated clubfeet

In 1981, Drs George Y. El Khory, Ernesto Ippolito, Stuart L. Weinstein, and myself evaluated the roentgenograms of 32 patients, 21 males and 11 females, with unilateral clubfoot deformity ranging in age from 14 to 32 years (average 20 years) (Ponseti *et al.* 1981). The clubfoot was treated with manipulation and plaster casts in eight of the patients and in 24 patients with a tenotomy of the tendo Achilles. There were ten relapses treated by further manipulation of the foot and transfer of the tibialis anterior tendon to the third cuneiform. Roentgenographic examination of the feet consisted of an anteroposterior standing view of 24 degrees cephalad angulation and lateral standing views(Templeton *et al.* 1965).

Using the normal foot as a control, the parameters listed below were evaluated in both feet and the data obtained was subjected to computer analysis. The paired *t*-test was used to assess statistical significance of the findings.

Tibia. On the lateral roentgenograms of the clubfeet but not in any of the normal feet, posterior slanting of the articular surface of the tibia was observed in 13 patients (39 per cent), and notching of the anterior lip of the distal tibia in 20 patients (63 per cent) (Fig. 52).

Talus. In the clubfeet, the length of the talus ranged from 4.3 to 6.1 cm (mean, 5.4 cm). In the normal feet, it ranged from 4.3 to 6.8 cm (mean 5.7). This difference is statistically significant ($t = 6.87$). Mild to moderate degrees of diminished convexity of the talar dome were observed in the lateral roentgenograms of 18 out of 32 clubfeet (56 per cent), but in all cases the curve of the trochlea was congruous with that of the articular surface of the tibia. There were no moderate or severe degrees of flat–top talus (Dunn and Samuelson 1974). Anteroposterior roentgenograms of 12 clubfeet (37 per cent) showed that the talar head was moderately flat in eight feet and dome–shaped in four (Fig. 53). In each patient, the angle of the neck with the body of the talus in the clubfoot was similar to that in the normal foot in the anteroposterior and lateral roentgenograms. On the lateral roentgenograms, the talar tubercle was small in 18 clubfeet (56 per cent), when compared with the opposite normal feet (Fig. 55).

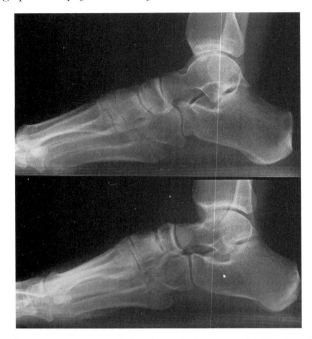

Fig. 52 Lateral roentgenograms of the feet of a 25-year-old female with right clubfoot deformity treated with five plaster casts during early infancy. At eight years of age, the deformity was relapsing and was treated by a transfer of the tibialis anterior tendon to the third cuneiform. At present, her functional rating is 94. On the clubfoot site (*bottom*), there is notching of the anterior lip of the tibia. The talar dome is not as spherical as in the normal foot (*top*). In the clubfoot, the head and lateral tubercle of the talus are small; the navicular is flat and the distance between the medial tubercle of the navicular and the medial malleolus is less than on the normal side.

Navicular. The navicular was wedge-shaped in 17 clubfeet (53 per cent), and flattened in 13 clubfeet (40 per cent). The medial displacement of the navicular was seen in the majority of the clubfeet. The navicular-medial malleolus distance in the clubfeet ranged from 0.7 cm to 2.9 cm (mean 1.4 cm); in the normal feet it ranges from 1.8 to 3.0 cm (mean 2.4 cm). This distance is statistically significant ($t = 9.2$) (Fig. 52). Mild dorsal displacement was also noted on the lateral roentgenograms in 11 clubfeet (34 per cent).

Calcaneus. The length of the calcaneus in the clubfeet ranged from 6.5 to 8.8 cm (mean, 7.6 cm), and in the normal feet from 6.8 to 9.1 cm (mean 7.8 cm). The difference is statistically significant ($t = 3.37$). On the anteroposterior roentgenograms the cuboid in the clubfeet was abducted in front of the calcaneus by a mean angle of 4.15 degrees while in the normal feet the mean angle was 2.13 degrees. The difference is not statistically significant ($t = 1.92$).

Cuneiforms. The cuneiforms were laterally displaced and angulated in front of the navicular in 19 clubfeet but not in the normal feet. The degree of angular

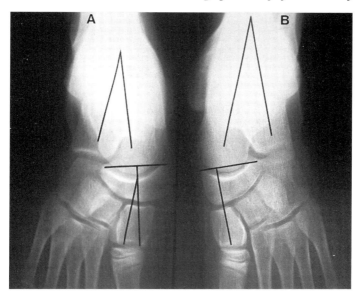

Fig. 53 Anteroposterior roentgenograms of the feet of a 13-year-old male with right clubfoot treated since birth with five plaster casts and percutaneous tendo Achilles tenotomy. His current functional rating is 98. In the clubfoot (A) the navicular is medially displaced in relation to the head of the talus and is seen to approximate the medial malleolus; the talar head is dome-shaped. The cuneiforms are laterally displaced and laterally angulated in relation to the navicular. The navicular–first cuneiform angle measures −14 degrees on the clubfoot and 0 degrees on the normal foot (B). The talo-calcaneal angle measures 20 degrees on the clubfoot and 23 degrees on the normal foot.

displacement of the cuneiforms was determined by the navicular–first cuneiform angle. To construct this angle a line was drawn through the long axis of the first cuneiform and another line was drawn perpendicular to the transverse axis of the navicular (Fig. 53). A negative value signifies abduction of the cuneiform. The navicular–first cuneiform angle in the clubfeet ranged from −53 to 0 degrees (mean, −17 degrees); in the normal feet it ranges from −17 to +13 degrees (mean, −1.7 degrees). The difference is statistically significant ($t = 6.76$).

Metatarsals. The length of the first metatarsal in the clubfeet ranged from 5.3 to 7.6 cm (mean, 6.54 cm) and in the normal feet from 5.5 to 7.9 cm (mean 6.58 cm). The difference is not statistically significant ($t = 0.6$). The length of the fifth metatarsal in the clubfeet ranged from 5.5 to 9.4 cm (mean, 7.35 cm); in the normal feet it ranged from 5.5 to 9.4 cm (mean, 7.37 cm). The difference is not statistically significant ($t = 0.51$).

Foot alignment. The talar–first metatarsal angle in the clubfeet ranged from −10 to +33 degrees (mean, +3.28 degrees); in the normal feet it ranged from −20 to +11 degrees (mean, −3.37 degrees). The difference is statistically significant ($t = 3.3$). The calcaneus fifth metatarsal angle in the clubfeet ranged

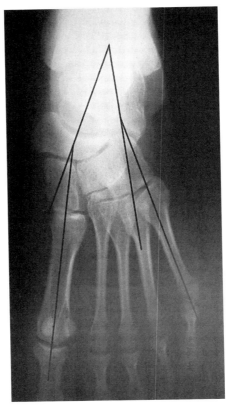

Fig. 54. Anteroposterior roentgenogram of a clubfoot in a 20-year-old female showing the calcaneus–fifth metatarsal and the talus—first metatarsal angles. These angles were used to determine the hindfoot–forefoot alignment. Both angles measure −12 degrees, degrees indicating a mild degree of abduction of the forefoot in relation to the hindfoot. The navicular is medially displaced and is wedge-shaped.

from −20 to +20 degrees (mean −4 degrees), in the normal feet from −18 to +5 degrees (mean, −3.37 degrees). This difference is not significant ($t = 0.49$) (Fig. 54).

Other observations. In the lateral roentgenograms, the distance between the posterior lip of the distal tibia and the opposing superior aspect of the calcaneus in the clubfeet ranged from 1.1 cm to 2.6 cm (mean, 1.76 cm), and in the normal feet it ranged from 1.3 cm to 2.9 cm (mean, 2.02 cm). The difference is statistically significant ($t = 4.58$) (Fig. 55).

Cavus was observed in only 4 of the 32 clubfeet with the first–fifth metatarsal angle on the lateral roentgenograms ranging from 17 to 39 degrees (mean, 27.7 degrees) on the lateral roentgenograms. In the other 28 clubfeet and in the normal feet, the mean was 12 degrees.

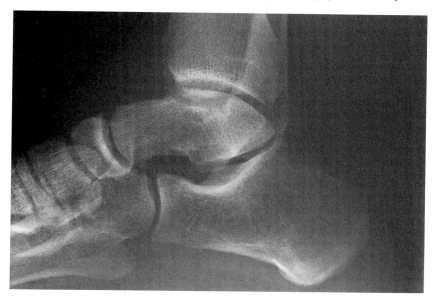

Fig. 55 Lateral roentgenogram of the clubfoot showing posterior slanting of the articulating surface of the tibia. The sphericity of the talar dome is diminished. The subtalar joint is markedly abnormal with continuous posterior and middle facets. There are no demonstrable anterior facets. The sinus tarsi is wide and the head of the talus is small.

In the clubfeet, the talocalcaneal angle on the anteroposterior roentgenogram ranged from 4 to 25 degrees (mean 15.7 degrees), and in the normal feet from 13 to 29 degrees (mean 20.7 degrees). This difference is statistically significant ($t = 6.3$) (Fig. 53). The talocalcaneal angle in the clubfeet on the lateral roentgenogram ranged from 10 to 34 degrees (mean, 23.1 degree), and in the normal feet from 17 to 46 degrees (mean, 31.6 degrees). This difference is statistically significant ($t = 6.1$). The talocalcaneal index in the clubfeet ranged from 16 to 51 degrees (mean, 37.7 degrees); in the normal feet it ranged from 37 to 64 degrees (mean, 52.3 degrees). This difference is statistically significant ($t = 8.57$).

Abnormalities in the size and configuration of the subtalar facet joints evidenced in 16 clubfeet were better delineated with the use of special views and computerized tomography. The posterior joint was small in size and slightly laterally slanted downwards, and the joint cartilage was of uneven thickness in some cases. The middle joint was small and sometimes merged with the posterior joint. The anterior joint was absent in most feet. The sinus tarsi was larger in the clubfoot (Fig. 55 and Figs 56A and 56B).

In a study of the long-term outcome of metatarsus adductus Farsetti *et al.* (1994) observed that in 68 per cent of their patients the profile of the first cuneiform–first metatarsal joint was in a posteromedially inclined plane. The

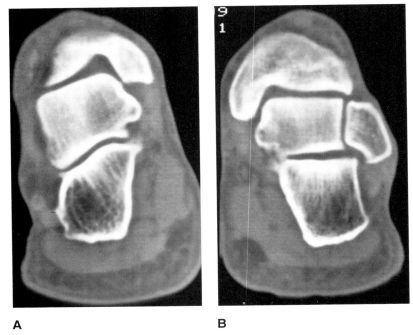

A   **B**

Figs 56A and 56B CT frontal sections of the hindfoot of two 38-year-old patients with treated clubfeet in infancy. The posterior subtalar joint in A is slanted laterally downwards. The thickness of the subtalar joint space in B is uneven.

alignment of this joint was studied on the roentgenograms of 114 treated clubfeet in 64 adult patients. The joint profile in the AP roentgenogram was close to perpendicular (90-degree angle) to the long axis of the first cuneiforms in 98 feet and it was moderately inclined (average 75-degree angle) in 16 feet (14 per cent). This observation suggests the presence of metatarsus adductus in some patients with clubfoot. (see Fig. 46G, Chapter 7).

Dynamic studies. In 10 patients, dynamics of both feet were studied employing fluoroscopy to determine the range and type of motion of the ankle, subtalar, and midtarsal joints. The posterior tibiocalcaneal distance measured on the lateral spot films, taken with the feet in maximum plantar flexion, was the same in the clubfoot as in the normal foot; however, in maximum dorsiflexion the posterior tibiocalcaneal distance was greater in the normal foot and, in some patients was even five times greater. The degree of dorsiflexion of the ankle, therefore, was greatly restricted in the clubfeet.

When supinating the clubfoot, the degree of adduction motion of the calcaneus under the talus was comparable to that of a normal foot. However, when pronating the clubfoot, the abduction of the calcaneus beyond a neutral position was restricted. The range of motion of the navicular was even more restricted. With pronation, the navicular-medial malleolar distance increases much more in a normal foot than in a clubfoot. The degree of heel valgus and foot pronation in the treated clubfeet was also restricted. The mobility of the cuboid and the mobility between the navicular and the cuneiforms in the clubfeet was not restricted as compared with the mobility in the normal feet.

In the spot films obtained during fluoroscopy, the degree of sliding or of scissoring motion between the talus and the calcaneus in the subtalar joint of the clubfeet was comparable to that of the normal feet when supinated; however, when the feet were pronated, the gliding of the calcaneus under the talus was greatly restricted in the clubfeet. The range of ankle dorsiflexion and subtalar motion was more restricted in the feet with functional results of less than 90 points with the talocalcaneal angle under 16 degrees than in the feet with functional ratings greater than 90 points.

Some of the residual abnormalities in treated clubfeet found in adults are remnants of the treatment and some are reminiscent of the anomalies present in the clubfeet of fetuses and newborns. The notching in the anterior lip and the posterior slant of the distal tibia appear to be related to the tight ligaments and tendons in the posterior and medial aspects of the ankle and subtalar joints. These tight structures limit dorsiflexion and pronation of the heel. The talar head is consequently prevented from sliding downward between the navicular and the sustentaculum, thereby exerting excessive pressure on the anterior lip of the tibia and stunting bone growth in the surrounding area. Similar compressive forces applied to the dome of the talus can result in its diminished convexity. In addition, the total length of the talus was significantly shorter in the clubfeet, thereby increasing the chance of contact between the neck of the talus and the anterior lip of the tibia.

The subtalar joint anomalies seen in the radiographic studies of adults were observed by us in sections obtained from clubfeet of fetuses (Ippolito and Ponseti 1980) as well as observed by other researchers in infants (Schlicht 1963; Waisbrod 1973; Simons 1977). These findings lead us to conclude that the size and configuration of the subtalar joint facets are determined in fetal life and that treatment will not alter them. Moreover, the restricted motion observed at the subtalar joint in clubfeet following treatment results not only from the short ligaments and tendons but also from the abnormal size and configuration of the articular facets in the joint.

Severe lateral rotation of the ankle with posterior displacement of the fibula described by some authors (Swann *et al.* 1969) did not occur in our patients except to a mild degree during the first years of our treatment. Although many of our treated clubfeet had small talocalcaneal angles and a medially displaced navicular, the heel varus was well corrected and the proper hindfoot–forefoot alignment was obtained by angling and shifting the cuneiforms laterally along with a slight increase in the lateral angulation of the cuboid.

The roentgenograms obtained in the 1993 follow-up study revealed skeletal changes similar to those observed in the roentgenograms of the same patients taken 16 years earlier. Degenerative changes consisting of some osteophytes on the dorsal aspect of the neck of the talus, the anterior distal tibia, and at the talonavicular joint were not increased except in two patients whose osteophytes on the talar neck were slightly larger. No narrowing of the joints or other signs of degenerative arthritis were observed.

References

Dunn, H.K. and Samuelson, K.M. (1974). Flat top talus. A long-term report of 20 clubfeet. *J. Bone Joint Surg.*, **56A**, 57.

Farsetti, P., Weinstein, S.L., and Ponseti, I.V. (1994). The long-term functional and radiographic outcomes of untreated and non-operatively treated metatarsus adductus. *J. Bone Joint Surg.*, **76A**, 257.

Ippolito, E. and Ponseti I.V. (1980). Congenital clubfoot in the human fetus. A histological study. *J. Bone Joint Surg.*, **62A**, 8.

Ponseti, I.V., El-Khoury, G.Y., Ippolito, E., and Weinstein, S. (1981). A radiographic study of skeletal deformities in treated clubfeet. *Clin. Orthop.*, **160**, 30.

Schlicht, D. (1963). The pathological anatomy of talipes equinovarus. Australian and New Zealand. *J. Surg.*, **33**, 2.

Simons, G.W. (1977). External rotational deformities in the clubfeet. *Clin. Orthop.*, **126**, 339.

Swann, M., Lloyd-Roberts, G.C., and Catterall, A. (1969). The anatomy of uncorrected clubfeet. A study of rotation deformity. *J. Bone Joint Surg.*, **51B**, 263.

Templeton, A.W., Mcalister, W.H., and Zim, I.D. (1965). Standardization of terminology and evaluation of osseous relationships in congenitally abnormal feet. *Am. J. Roentgenol.*, **93**, 374.

Waisbrod, H. (1973). Congenital clubfoot: An anatomical study. *J. Bone Joint Surg.*, **55B**, 796.

11
Errors in treatment

To avoid most errors in treatment, orthopedists must understand three basic features of the clubfoot:

- Although the whole foot is in extreme supination, the hindfoot is much more firmly held in adduction and inversion by tight ligaments and tendons than the forefoot. Indeed, most joint ligaments in the forefoot are normal at birth and usually the forefoot is supple and not as supinated as the hindfoot.
- The calcaneus, the navicular and the cuboid are severely medially displaced as well as inverted. The medial displacement and inversion of all three bones are corrected by first abducting the foot in supination under the talus. Then gradually reducing the supination to a neutral position while the foot is further abducted. The main corrective manipulation of the clubfoot, therefore, is foot abduction. Attempts to pronate the foot beyond its neutral position is a very common and pernicious maneuver.
- An anatomical reduction of all the skeletal elements of the clubfoot is not feasible, nor is it indispensable for a well-aligned foot with good long-lasting functional results.

The delicate task of manipulating clubfeet and applying plaster casts cannot be delegated to unsupervised assistants. This task should be performed by an experienced orthopedic surgeon who knows the pathological anatomy of the deformity and the proper corrective manipulative technique applied in the first few months of life. If this initial treatment is faulty, the correction not only fails but the deformity is compounded, and the clubfoot is made stiffer and much more difficult or even impossible to correct.

The most frequent errors in the manipulative treatment of clubfeet are:

1. Everting the forefoot rather than supinating and abducting it. Forefoot eversion causes an increase of the cavus which becomes rigid as the plantar fascia thickens and tightens (see Fig. 27, Chapter 7).
2. Attempts to correct foot supination by forcefully pronating the foot. This causes a breach in the midfoot because the calcaneus remains locked in inversion by the tight medial tarsal ligaments.
3. Attempts to externally rotate the foot while the heel in fixed in varus.

This causes a posterior displacement of the lateral malleolus by externally rotating the talus in the ankle joint. The posterior displacement of the lateral malleolus is an iatrogenic deformity. It does not occur when the foot is abducted in flexion and slight supination to stretch the tibio-navicular and calcaneonavicular ligaments thereby allowing the calcaneus to abduct under the talus and the heel varus to correct.

4. Attempts to correct foot adduction by abducting the forefoot against pressure at the calcaneocuboid joint (Kite's error). This blocks the abduction of the calcaneus and the reduction of the cuboid subluxation. Furthermore, the ligaments at the Lisfranc line are stretched and weakened hampering correction of the hindfoot (see Fig. 28, Chapter 7).

5. Attempts to correct heel varus by everting the calcaneus without first abducting (externally rotating) the calcaneus under the talus.

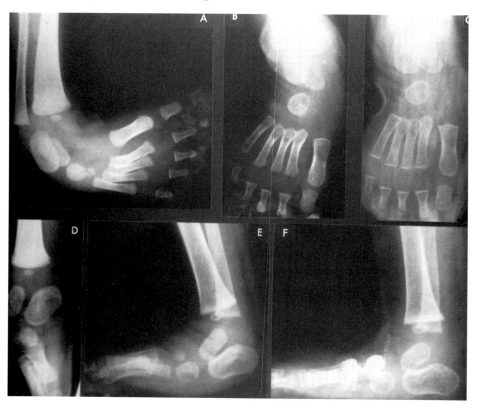

A

Fig. 57A These roentgenograms of a patient with clubfeet illustrate the development of a rocker-botton deformity resulting from attempts to correct the equinus by dorsiflexing the forefoot. The cuboid remained medially displaced. The deformity was improved by lengthening the tendo Achilles. At 6 years of age the patient had a transfer of the tibialis anterior tendon to the third cuneiform.

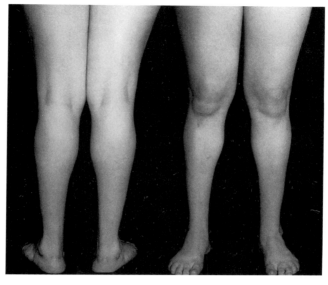

B

Fig. 57B At 26 years of age the feet look normal. The calves are small and the patient has some foot pain after walking more than two miles.

6. Applications of below-the-knee plaster casts instead of toe-to-groin casts; the latter are needed to prevent the ankle and talus from rotating. Since the foot must be held in abduction under the talus, the talus must not rotate. Otherwise, the correction obtained by manipulation is lost.

7. Attempts to correct the equinus before the other components of the deformity are corrected. A rocker-bottom deformity will result preventing correction of the heel varus (Fig. 57).

8. Attempts to correct the equinus by dorsiflexing the forefoot instead of the whole foot, thereby causing a rocker-bottom deformity.

9. Prolonged plaster-cast immobilization of the foot for three or more weeks between manipulations. This results in osteoporosis and in excessive loosening of the normal ligaments in front of the navicular and cuboid, thereby weakening the lever arm formed by the anterior part of the foot, needed for the correction of the tarsal deformities.

10. Prolonged immobilization for many months and rough manipulations. This causes stunting of the tibial growth plates and results in leg shortening.

11. Frequent manipulations not followed by immobilization. Such manipulations are ineffective. The foot must be immobilized with the contracted ligaments at the maximum stretch obtained after each manipulation.

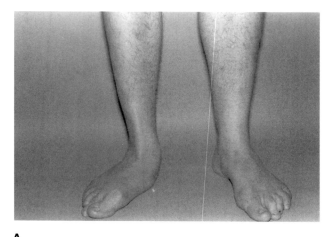

A

B

Figs 58A and 58B This 36-year-old patient was born with bilateral congenital clubfeet treated with manipulations and plaster casts in infancy. At 6 years of age the feet looked normal but the mother was told by the doctor after seeing the roentgenograms that surgery was necessary to improve the position of the bones. The mother consented to the operation in one foot only. A posteromedial release was done on the right foot. After surgery the foot became stiff and progressively flattened. Now the patient has much pain in the operated foot and very little motion in the mid-tarsal joints. A triple arthrodesis has been indicated. The left foot is painless and well aligned.

Plaster casts applied between manipulations serve two purposes: (1) to keep the ligaments stretched, and (2) to loosen them sufficiently to facilitate further stretching in the following manipulations at intervals of 5 to 7 days.

12. Attempts to obtain a perfect anatomical correction of the displaced navicular in very severe clubfoot deformities in infants. In such cases, foot ad-

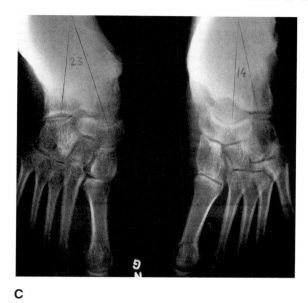

C

Fig. 58C The talocalcaneal angle measures 23 degrees in the right foot and only 14 degrees in the left. The navicular is well aligned in the right foot and medially displaced in the left. However, the talonavicular joint space is very narrow in the right and normal in the left.

duction and heel varus can often be corrected by manipulation, without radical surgery, by abducting the cuneiforms in front of the partially reduced navicular and by abducting the cuboid in front of the calcaneus, in addition to transferring the tibialis anterior tendon to the third cuneiform. This 'spurious' correction is compatible with a fully functional, well-aligned foot. Only few very severe, stiff, unyielding clubfeet will need to be corrected surgically (Fig. 58).

13. Failure to use shoes attached to a bar in external rotation full-time for three months and at night for several years until retracting fibrosis and overpull of the tibialis posterior muscle abate.

14. Transfer of the tibialis anterior tendon to the fifth metatarsal or to the cuboid. An excessive foot eversion may result.

15. Pulling the tibialis anterior tendon out of its compartment under the superior extensor retinaculum before the tendon is transferred. The tendon will bowstring forward in front of the ankle.

16. Splitting the tibialis anterior tendon to insert only half of it to the lateral aspect of the foot. This procedure causes dorsiflexion of the foot but does not correct foot supination. To correct foot supination the tendon must be transferred to the third cuneiform.

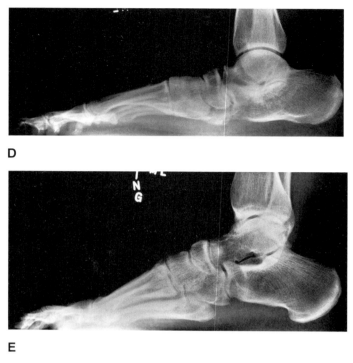

D

E

Figs 58D and 58E The right foot (D) is very flat and the subtalar joint space is very narrow. Spurs are present in the dorsal aspect of the talar head. In the left foot the subtalar joint has an abnormal configuration but its joint space is well preserved.

Index